ABC of MEDICINE
(with Mnemonics)

ABC of MEDICINE
(with Mnemonics)

Sixteenth Edition

Aspi F Golwalla
MD FACC FCPS FCCP
Emeritus Professor
Department of Medicine
GS Medical College and KEM Hospital
Mumbai, Maharashtra, India

Sharukh A Golwalla
MD (Med) DM (Card) FCCP
(Specialized in Echocardiography)
Cardiologist
Breach Candy Hospital, Jaslok Hospital
Sir HN Reliance Foundation Hospital
Mumbai, Maharashtra, India

JAYPEE

JAYPEE BROTHERS MEDICAL PUBLISHERS
The Health Sciences Publisher
New Delhi | London

Jaypee Brothers Medical Publishers (P) Ltd

Headquarters
EMCA House, 23/23-B Ansari Road,
Daryaganj New Delhi 110 002, India
Landline: +91-11-23272143,
+91-11-23272703
+91-11-23282021, +91-11-23245672
e-mail: jaypee@jaypeebrothers.com

Corporate Office
4838/24, Ansari Road,
Daryaganj New Delhi 110 002, India
Phone: +91-11-43574357
Fax: +91-11-43574314
e-mail: jaypee@jaypeebrothers.com

Overseas Office
JP Medical Ltd.
83, Victoria Street, London
SW1H 0HW (UK)
Phone: +44-20 3170 8910
e-mail: info@jpmedpub.com

EU GPSR Authorised Representative
Logos Europe, 9 rue Nicolas Poussin
17000, La Rochelle, France
Phone: +33 (0) 6 67 93 73 78
e-mail: contact@logoseurope.eu

Website: www.jaypeebrothers.com
Website: www.jaypeedigital.com

ABC of Medicine (with Mnemonics)
Sixteenth Edition: 2020
Reprint: 2026
ISBN 978-93-86150-75-2
Printed in India

Preface

We are happy to present the sixteenth edition of this handbook especially for the undergraduate medical students in various faculties, usually Allopathy and Homeopathy.

The text has been updated with additional contents. The contents include all the Chapters systemwise as well as a miscellaneous Chapter to make it all inclusive.

As before, we would like to quote the age old dictum. "If you refuse to remember mnemonics, you will fail and be happy as chronics."

Once again, suggestions for good additional 'mugging' are looked forward to 2020.

Aspi F Golwalla
Sharukh A Golwalla

Contents

CHAPTER

Gastrointestinal, Liver and Biliary Tract

1

VOMITING

Causes

1. Abdominal
   Gastric: Gastritis, food poisoning, pyloric stenosis.
   Extragastric: Viral hepatitis. Appendicitis, renal or biliary colic, intestinal obstruction, etc.
2. **B**rain: Raised intracranial pressure, tumor, Meniere's
3. **C**ardiac: Myocardial infarction, congestive heart failure (CHF)
4. **D**rugs: **D**igitalis
5. **E**ndocrine and metabolic: Diabetic ketoacidosis, pregnancy
6. **F**unctional or **PRO:**
   - **P**ain-induced: Peptic ulcer, acute appendicitis
   - **R**eflex: Meningitis, uremia, diabetic ketoacidosis
   - **O**bstructive: Esophageal, intestinal.

CONSTIPATION

Acute

- **A**ppendicitis, (acute)
- **B**owel obstruction
- **C(S)**ystemic illness
- **D**ehydration.

Chronic

Anorexia nervosa (and other psychiatric illness, e.g. depression)

Bowel disease: Ca, irritable bowel syndrome (IBS), ulcerative colitis (UC), Crohn's

Central nervous system (CNS) lesions:

Peripheral: Hirschsprung's, autonomic neuropathy

Central: Cerebrovascular accident (CVA), Parkinson's, multiple sclerosis (MS)

Muscular: Dermatomyositis, systemic sclerosis

Drugs: Codeine, anticholinergics, antidepressives

Endocrine: Diabetes mellitus (DM), hypothyroidism, hypercalcemia.

Faulty habits: Laxative abuse

Geriatrics: Old age

Hemorrhoids and other anorectal disorders

Insufficient fiber in diet.

DIARRHEA

Acute

- Allergic
- Bacterial (or viral) food poisoning
- Chemicals and toxins, e.g. mushroom, sea food
- Drugs: Amoxycillin, colchicin.

Chronic

Infections: Giardia, *E. histolytica*, AIDS
Inadequate absorption: Chronic pancreatitis, short bowel syndrome, bacterial overgrowth
Iatrogenic: Drugs
Intolerance, e.g. lactose
Inflammatory bowel disease
Ingestion (excess): Fructose, sorbitol, caffeine, purgatives
Infiltration: Pancreatic Ca, gastrinoma, carcinoid
Idiopathic secretory diarrhea
Incontinence (fecal) and
Metabolic: Diabetes mellitus, hyperthyroidism, hyperadrenalism.

ACUTE ABDOMEN

Causes

A. **Intra-abdominal:**
Appendicitis, acute mesenteric lymphadenitis, aneurysm (dissecting)

Burst (perforation): Peptic ulcer
Colic: Biliary, ureteric, volvulus of sigmoid, torsion of ovarian cyst
Dysentery
Enterocolitis
Factitious
Growth: Cecum, right colon
Hemorrhage: Rupture of spleen, ruptured ectopic pregnancy
Inflammation: Acute cholecystitis, acute pancreatitis
Ischemic: Acute mesenteric ischemia.

B. **Extra-abdominal:**
Chest: Acute pulmonary or pleural infection
CNS: Herpes (lower thoracic)
Crisis: Hemolytic, porphyria, tabetic
C(K)etoacidosis: Diabetic.

Children:
- Infection of urinary tract
- Intussusception.

UPPER ABDOMINAL PAIN

Causes

A. **Extra-abdominal:**
1. Chest:
Heart: Angina, infarction
Lungs: Infarction, pleurisy

Nerves: Herpes zoster
Bones: Fracture rib, spinal tumor.
2. **C**risis: Hemolytic anemia, tabes, lead poisoning, acute porphyria.
3. **C(K)**etoacidosis: Diabetic.

B. **Abdominal:**
1. Trauma to abdominal wall or organ
2. Hollow organ disease:
Stomach: Peptic ulcer, hiatus hernia, gastritis
Gallbladder: Cholelithiasis, cholecystitis
Intestine: Bowel obstruction
Aorta: Aneurysm.
Renal pelvis or ureter: Calculus, clot.
3. Solid organ disease:
Liver: Inflammation, tumor
Pancreas: Pancreatitis, tumor
Kidney: Stone, inflammation, tumor
Spleen: Infarct.

RECURRENT ABDOMINAL PAIN WITH NEGATIVE TESTS

Pancreatitis
Porphyria
Psychiatric disorder.

STOMATITIS

Aphthous
Allergic

B-complex deficiency
Catarrhal
Drug-induced
Erythema multiforme (and other skin diseases, e.g. lichen planus)
Fungal.

BURNING MOUTH: 4Ds

Dermatological condition: Lichen planus, candidosis and other infections
Depression (Psychogenic)
Deficiency: Iron, folate, B_{12}
Drugs: Captopril.

GINGIVAL SWELLING

Systemic Causes

Amyloidosis
Blood diseases: Leukemia
Crohn's disease
Deficiency: Scurvy
Endocrine: Pregnancy
Fibromatosis (hereditary gingival)
Granulomatosis (Wegener's)
Hurler's syndrome
Iatrogenic: Phenytoin, cyclosporin, nifedipine, diltiazem.

LEUKOPLAKIA

Sepsis
Smoking
Spices
Spirits
Sharp teeth
Syphilis and HIV infection

DYSPHAGIA

1. **Oropharyngeal:**

Symptoms:	*Lesion:*
Difficulty in initiating swallowing	Functional, XI nerve lesion, motor neuron disease
Coughing, choking, nasal regurgitation	Upper motor neuron: Bilateral hemiplegia Multiple sclerosis
Lump in throat	Pharyngeal pouch, thyroid, postcricoid, psychosomatic (Globus hystericus pharyngeus)

2. **Esophageal:**

Symptoms:	*Lesion:*
Hold up of food in chest Worse with solids	**Mechanical block—** *In lumen:* Foreign body *In wall:* Stricture, Ca. Plummer-Vinson *Outside wall:* Aneurysm, neoplasm.

Liquids and solids	**Motor dysfunction—** Achalasia, spasm, systemic sclerosis
Chest pain on swallowing	Esophagitis, spasm, achalasia

HEMATEMESIS

Esophagus: Esophagitis, growth, foreign body
Esophagogastric junction: Varices, Mallory-Weiss tear

1. *Ulcer:* Chronic duodenal, chronic gastric
2. *Gastric erosions:* Aspirin, alcohol
3. *Hiatus hernia*
4. *Miscellaneous:* Ca stomach, bleeding disorder, hereditary telangiectasia, portal hypertension, gastropathy.

GASTROESOPHAGEAL REFLUX DISEASE (GERD)

Clinical Features

Gastric: Heartburn, dysphagia, chest pain, water brash, globus sensation
Pulmonary: Chronic cough, post-nasal drip, sore throat, coughing spells
Miscellaneous: Sleep disturbance due to nocturnal reflux.

Management

Phase I (Mild symptoms): Raising head end of bed, antacids, dinner 2 hours before bed time
Phase II: H_2 receptor blockers or PPI if no response
Phase III: Proton pump inhibitor. Prokinetic drugs.

HIATUS HERNIA

Types

- Sliding (90%)
- Rolling.

Clinical Features

1. **A**cid reflux: Dysphagia, heartburn, retrosternal discomfort
2. **B**leeding
3. **C**hest symptoms: Cough, anginal pains, palpitation
4. **D**iseases associated: Peptic ulcer, gallstones.

PEPTIC ULCER

Pathogenesis

Anxiety
Burns
Cigarette smoking
Drug-induced

Endocrine [Hyperparathyroidism syndrome (Zollinger Ellison syndrome)]
Family history
Gastric acidity (No acid, no ulcer)
Higher incidence (Cirrhosis, Cushing's)
Infection (*Helicobacter pylori*).

Symptoms

Pain

Site: Epigastric
Character and severity: Continuous boring, mild to severe
Onset: Gradual
Periodicity: Remissions
Radiation: To back if penetrating ulcer
Aggravation: FAST
- **F**atty food, fatigue
- **A**lcohol
- **S**pices
- **T**ension

Relief: Food, vomiting, antacids
Special feature: No pain on rising in morning
Associated symptoms: Water brash, heartburn.

Complications

In addition to bleeding:
Pyloric stenosis
Perforation
Penetration

Management

Medical

Avoidance of: Alcohol, tobacco, spicy and greasy food
Bed rest: **D**uring acute phase
Control of anxiety: Tranquilizers, psychotherapy
Drugs:

1. Acid suppression by:
   Antacids
   Anticholinergics
   Antagonists (H_2 receptor)
   ATPase proton pump inhibitor compounds (e.g. Omeprazole)
2. Anti-*H. pylori* agents
3. A(E)nhancement of mucosal defense factors: Sucralfate.

Surgical

Indications for Surgery in DU

Pyloric stenosis
Perforation
Penetrating ulcer
Persistent pain
Profuse (or recurrent) bleeding
Probability of malignancy
Poor patient (Economic consideration).

ABDOMINAL LUMP

Examine for

Situation
Size
Shape
Surface
Skin overlying (including temp.)
Softness (fluctuation)
Sensitivity (tenderness)
Shifting (mobility)
Spread
Stethoscopy (bruit)

Lump in Right Iliac Fossa

Appendicular mass
Bacillus (Koch's) infection
Crohn's disease, carcinoid
Diverticular disease
Ectopic kidney
Fungal (Actinomycosis)
Growth (Ca cecum)
Histolytica infection (Ameboma)

Lump in Left Iliac Fossa

Adenopathy (Inguinal)
Bowel lumps (Fecal)
Crohn's disease
Diverticulitis
Ectopic (or transplanted) kidney
Follicular (Ovarian) cysts
Growth

ABDOMINAL TUBERCULOSIS

Site	Lesion	Clinical Features
Small intestine	Ulcerative	Diarrhea, malabsorption, low GI bleeding
	Stricture	Intestinal obstruction + **P**erforation **P**eritonitis **P**yrexia **P**urging **P**oor absorption
Ileocecum and large intestine	Hypertrophic	Intestinal obstruction Mass
	Ulcero-hypertrophic	Lower GI bleed Fever
Peritoneum	Ascitic	Fluid, fever
	Adhesive	Intestinal obstruction
Mesenteric lymph-adenitis	Lymph nodes	Abdominal pain Fever Weight loss

MALABSORPTION SYNDROME

Causes

1. **Mucosal diseases:** Celiac disease, tropical sprue, parasitic infection (helminths, giardia), HIV illness

2. **Abnormal bacterial activity:** Intestinal TB, post-gastrectomy, Crohn's disease
3. **Pancreatic insufficiency:** Tropical pancreatitis
4. **Lymphatic obstruction:** Intestinal lymphangiectasia, blockage due to lymph nodes
5. **Genetic transmitted disorder:** Abetalipoproteinemia, fructose or lactose malabsorption.

Investigations: 3 Bs

1. **Biochemical:**
   Absorption of vitamin B_{12}
   (<8% urinary excretion in 48 hours)
   Breath test (For bacterial overgrowth)
   C(S)ecretin test: For pancreatic function
   D-xylose absorption (25 g oral)
   5 hr urinary excretion >4.5 g
   Electrolytes: and serum levels of
   vitamin B_{12}, iron, folic acid, calcium, albumin
   Fat in stool >6 g/24 h
   Glucose tolerance
2. **Barium meal:** Flocculation
   Feathery pattern
   (Also X-rays of chest and abdomen)
3. **Biopsy:** (Endoscopy small intestinal): Mucosal atrophy in celiac disease.

Results of Malabsorption

Fat	Steatorrhea, weight loss
Carbohydrate	Flatulent dyspepsia, abdominal distension
Protein	Edema, wasting
Vitamins	
A	Follicular hyperkeratosis Nyctalopia Bitot spots Xerophthalmia
B_1	Beriberi Fluid retention Brainstem lesion Wernicke's encephalopathy
B_2	Angular stomatitis, cheilosis Purple (magenta) tongue Corneal vascularization Scrotal dermatitis
Nicotinic acid	Pellagra: **3Ds** **Diarrhea** **Dementia** **Dermatitis**

C	Petechial hemorrhages
	Swollen gums
	Hyperkeratosis
	Follicular congestion
D	Osteomalacia
	Proximal myopathy
	Rickets in children
K	Purpura, hemorrhages
Folic acid	Macrocytic anemia
Vitamin B_{12}	Macrocytic anemia
	Pigmentation
Trace Elements	
Iron	Microcytic anemia
Sodium	Muscular weakness, cramps
Potassium	Flaccidity, arrhythmias
Calcium	Paresthesiae
Magnesium	Tetany
Zinc	Acrodermatitis
	Poor wound healing
	Growth retardation
	Increased susceptibility to infections
	Cognitive impairment
	Defective taste
Bile salts	Watery diarrhea

Selenium	Osteoporosis, cardiac arrhythmia
Phosphate	Whitening of nail beds. Pseudoalbinism, peripheral neuropathy, myalgia
Chromium	Glucose intolerance
Copper	Menkes kinky hair disease, retarded growth, cerebral degeneration.

INFLAMMATORY BOWEL DISEASE

Ulcerative Colitis, Crohn's Disease

Clinical Features

Anemia
Bloody diarrhea
Cramps (before defecation)
Decreased weight
E(A)norexia
Fever

Extraintestinal Manifestations

Related to activity	*Not-related to activity*
Aphthous ulcer	Sacroiliitis
Arthritis (large joints)	Arthralgia (small joints)
Episcleritis	
Erythema nodosum	

Differential Diagnosis

	Ulcerative colitis	Crohn's disease
Clinical:		
Fever	In severe cases	Common
Abdominal pain	Uncommon	Common
Perianal disease	Rare	Common
Abdominal mass	No	Common
Rectal bleeding	Invariable	Uncommon
Strictures	Rare	Common
Fistulas	Very rare	May occur
Toxic megacolon	Occasional	Rare
Radiological:		
Distribution	Continuous	Segmental
Mucosa	Fine ulceration	'Rose thorn' ulcers
Appearance	String sign	Hose pipe
Histological:		
Distribution	Mucosal	Transmural
Cellular infiltrate	Neutrophils, eosinophils	Lymphocytes, macrophages
Glands	Destruction	Preserved
Special features	None	Granulomata Aphthous ulcers

Endoscopic:

Friability	Characteristic	May occur
Distribution	Continuous	Discontinuous

Management

Medical

SLZ and 5-ASA
Corticosteroids
Immunomodulator
Antibiotics/probiotics.

Surgery

Toxic megacolon, perforation, massive hemorrhage, colon cancer.

ACUTE DIVERTICULITIS

Clinical features of left-sided appendicitis.

RECTAL BLEEDING

Causes

Angiodysplasia (in elderly), adenomatous polyp
Bowel disease: Inflammatory
Colitis (Ischemic, Crohn's)
Diverticular disease (including Meckel's)
E(**I**)rradiation proctitis

Fissure (perianal)
Growth. "Gay bowel" syndrome, colonic polyps
Hemorrhoids
Iatrogenic: GI bleeding from drugs

LIVER FUNCTION TESTS

Investigation	Normal range	Abnormality
1. *Synthetic function*		
Albumin PT PTT	35–50 g/L 10–14 sec 32–42 sec	Lowered: Cirrhosis Prolonged: Cholestasis Hepatocellular damage
2. *Excretory*		
Total serum bilirubin Unconjugated	Up to 1.5 mg/L	Raised: > production– Hemolysis Failure of transport Gilbert's Crigler-Najjar
Conjugated		Raised: Failure of excretion Dubin-Johnson Roter Hepatocellular damage: Viral hepatitis, cirrhosis, cholestasis

Contd...

Contd...

Investigation	Normal range	Abnormality
3. *Cholestasis*		
Alkaline phosphatase	30–110 IU/L	Raised: Cholestasis Hepatic metastases hepatitis. CAH Alcoholic cirrhosis Primary biliary cirrhosis
4. *Liver cell damage* Aminotransferases		
GGT	0–65 IU/L	Raised: Acute
AST ALT	5–40 IU/L	Raised: Cholestasis Viral and drug-induced hepatitis Malignant liver disease Infectious mononucleosis
5. *Alpha-fetoprotein* (<20 ng/mL)		
Raised: **Ca** liver **Ca** stomach, pancreas, GB, bile ducts, lungs Chronic active hepatitis Cirrhosis Pregnancy		

LIVER BIOPSY

Indications

1. **Investigation of liver disease:**
   Suspected drug reaction

Chronic—Cirrhosis
Focal lesions—Liver tumors.

2. **Investigation of systemic disease:**
   PUO, lymphomas, sarcoidosis, amyloidosis, tuberculosis
3. **Assessment of progress:**
   Chronic active hepatitis
4. **Liver transplant assessment.**

Contraindications

Ascites (gross)
Biliary obstruction (extrahepatic)
Chronic passive congestion
Defective clotting
E(**I**)infection: in liver, peritoneum or biliary tract
Failure: Hepatocellular (if severe)
Glioma (Hemangioma)
Hydatid cyst
Inability to cooperate with breathing maneuvers.

Complications

Injury: Penetration of GB or major bile ducts or viscera
Hemorrhage from capsular tears
Infection: Cholangitis
Intrahepatic: A-V fistula or hemorrhage

ACUTE VIRAL HEPATITIS

Hepatitis	Transmission	Salient Features
A	Enteric	Fever, jaundice. Never causes liver disease
B	Parenteral	Acute liver disease with chronic disease
		Risk of hepatic Ca
C	Parenteral	Chronic liver disease with risk of hepatic Ca
D	Parenteral	Depends on HBV for replication and expression
E	Enteric	Acute self-limiting hepatitis
		No carrier state or chronic disease

CHRONIC HEPATITIS

Chronic HBV

Stages of Infection

	Phase 1	Phase 2	Phase 3	Phase 4
Viremia	HBV tolerance HBeAg +ve viremia	HBV elimination	Latent HBV	Emergence of HBV variant HBeAg –ve viremia

Liver histology	Chronic lobular hepatitis	Minimal hepatitis active hepatitis	Chronic lobular/ active hepatitis
	Chronic persis-tent	Cirrhosis	
	Inactive cirrhosis	Active cirrhosis	Hepato-cellular cancer

Conditions Associated with HBsAg Carrier State

Lepromatous leprosy
Leukemias
Hodgkin's disease
Hemodialysis (chronic)
HIV infection
Drug addicts (needle users)
Down's syndrome.

Major Immune Disorders of the Liver

Autoimmune hepatitis
Biliary cirrhosis (primary)
Cholangitis (primary sclerosing).

JAUNDICE

Classification

1. **Prehepatic:** Hemolysis
2. **Hepatocellular:** (Medical jaundice)
   Acute: Viral, drug, toxic, parasitic
   Chronic: Cirrhosis liver with failure
   Congenital hyperbilirubinemia.
3. **Posthepatic/Cholestatic:**
   a. *Intrahepatic:* Cellular
      Alcoholic hepatitis (Also viral)
      Biliary cirrhosis
      Cholangitis (Primary sclerosing)
      Drugs—Sex hormones, phenothiazines.
   b. *Extrahepatic:* Mechanical (Surgical jaundice)
      Inside duct: Gallstone, FB, parasite
      Duct wall: Atresia, neoplasm
      Outside wall: Ca head of pancreas or ampulla
      Pancreatitis. Metastasis in porta hepatis.

Summary of Diagnostic Features

Feature	Obstructive	Liver cell	Hemolytic
Depth	Mild-deep	Mild-deep	Mild
Pruritus	Marked	Transient	Nil
Urine	Dark	Dark	Normal

Contd...

Contd...

Feature	Obstructive	Liver cell	Hemolytic
Stool	Pale	Pale	Normal or dark
Positive LFTs	Alkaline phosphatase	Bilirubin	(Conjugation) high
	Bilirubin (Conjugation)	(Conjugation + Free) Transaminases	Free bilirubin (high)

CIRRHOSIS OF LIVER

Causes

Alcoholic liver disease
B-hepatitis: (Also HCV).
Congestive: Anemia (Sickle cell)
Budd-Chiari syndrome
CHF
Drugs: Methotrexate, amiodarone, oxyphenisatin, halothane.
E(I)diopathic (cryptogenic)
Familial
- Galactosemia
- Glycogenosis (Type IV)
- Hemochromatosis
- Hepatolenticular degeneration (Wilson's)
- Tyrosinemia
- α-antitrypsin deficiency

Gallbladder disease: Stone, biliary stricture.

Clinical Features

1. **Hepatocellular failure:**
   Alimentary: Jaundice, ascites, parotid enlargement
   Blood: Anemia, purpura
   Circulatory: Hyperdynamic circulation, A-V shunts
   Dermatological: Spider nevi, palmar erythema, Dupuytren's contracture, paper money skin
   Endocrine: Gynecomastia, alopecia, impotence, testicular atrophy
   Fetor hepaticus
   Flap
   F(Ph)eral (peri) neuritis.
2. **Portal hypertension:**
   Ascites
   Bleeding (hematemesis, piles)
   Caput Medusae (Prominent abdominal veins)
   Diminished liver size
   Enlarged spleen

   Special features of alcoholic cirrhosis: END

   Enlarged parotid
   Neuritis
   Dupuytren's contracture.

Complications: 7 Hs

Hematemesis
Hepatic encephalopathy
Hepatorenal syndrome

Hepatoma
Herniae
Hemorrhoids
(H)infection.

ASCITES

Causes of Ascites

Common: 5 Ps

Peritonitis (TB, malignant)
Portal hypertension (Cirrhosis)
Pump failure (CHF)
Protein deficiency or loss (Nephrosis)
Pericarditis (constrictive).

Uncommon

Aneurin deficiency
Biliary
Chylous
Dropsy (epidemic)
Endocrine: Myxedema
Female disorder: Ovarian (Meigs' syndrome), endometriosis, struma ovarii
Glandular: Pancreatic.

Hemorrhagic fluid	*Chylous fluid*
Trauma	Trauma to thoracic duct
Tuberculosis	Tuberculosis
Tumor	Tumor invading thoracic duct
Thrombosis of mesenteric artery	Thrombosis of subclavian vein
	Tropical disease (Filaria)

Ascites with Minimal Edema of Feet: 5 Cs

Constrictive pericarditis
Cirrhosis
Cardiomyopathy (Restrictive)
Cruveilhier-Baumgarten syndrome
C(**K**)och's peritonitis.

Cirrhotic ascites—Subtract concentration of ascitic fluid albumin from serum albumin; a serum ascites albumin gradient of >1.1 g/L predicts portal hypertension with great accuracy.

Causes of Abdominal Distension: 9 Fs.

Full bladder	Fat
Firm mass	Feces
(Spleen, kidney, liver, ovary)	Flatus
Fatal growths	Fetus
Fluid	False pregnancy

PRIMARY BILIARY CIRRHOSIS

Clinical Features

Predominantly in middle-aged females
Pigmentation (and xanthoma)
Persistent jaundice
Pruritus
Portal hypertension, ascites, variceal hemorrhages.

Diagnosis

Increased immunoglobulins (particularly IgM)
plus
Alkaline phosphatase
Alpha-glutamyl transferase
Antimitochondrial antibodies.

Associated Conditions

Malabsorption
Malignancy: Extrahepatic: Breast
Intrahepatic: Carcinoma
Miscellaneous autoimmune conditions: Sicca syndrome, thyroid disease, arthropathy, etc.

Drug Therapy

Based on histological progression of disease

1. **Immune-mediated bile duct damage:**
   Immunosuppressive drugs: Prednisolone, cyclosporin or methotrexate

2. **Cholestasis:** Choleretic agents, e.g. ursodeoxycholic acid
3. **Fibrosis:** Antifibrotics, e.g. colchicine.

ACUTE HEPATIC FAILURE

Causes: 5 Hs

1. **H**epatic disease
   Cirrhosis, viral hepatitis. Pregnancy (fatty liver)
2. **H**ypersensitivity to drugs: Isoniazid, Rifampicin. Diclofenac, ketoconazole. Tricyclic antidepressants. Antiepileptics
3. **H**alothane anesthesia
4. **H**igh dose paracetamol. Also mushroom poisoning
5. **H**ypoxic injury.

Clinical Features

Apraxia (Constructional)
Bad breath (Sweet, slightly fecal)
Confusion
Drowsiness (progressing to coma)
Enhanced tendon reflexes, muscle tone
Flapping tremors (liver flap).

Precipitating Factors of Hepatic Encephalopathy

Alcoholic bout
Bleeding
Constipation
Drugs: Sedatives

Electrolyte imbalance
Fluid tapping
Gastroenteritis (Diarrhea, vomiting)
High protein diet
Hypokalemia
Infection
Iatrogenic: Post-portosystemic shunt or TIPS.

Management of Fulminant Hepatic Failure

Hepatic encephalopathy	No proteins, bowel wash, Neomycin
	Lactulose
Hypoglycemia	IV glucose
Hemorrhage (GI)	Vasoactive drugs
	Balloon tamponade
	Endoscopic sclero-therapy or banding
	TIPS
	Surgery
Hyponatremia	Water restriction
Hypokalemia	IV supplements
Hypotension	Dopamine
Hypovolemia	Blood, plasma

Hyperventilation (Resp. alkalosis)	IV soda bicarbonate
Hepatorenal syndrome	Hemodialysis
High ICP	IV mannitol
H(I)nfection	Antibiotics
High risk	Liver transplant

LIVER TRANSPLANTATION

Indications

- Cirrhosis (decompensated)
- Acute liver failure
- Liver cancer.

Others

- Hepatic venous obstruction progressing to cirrhosis (treated unsuccessfully)
- Genetic disorder:
  Wilson's disease
  Crigler-Najjar syndrome.

Contraindications

AIDS
Behavior (chaotic–ongoing alcohol or substance abuse)
Cardiopulmonary disease (severe)

Disseminated malignancy
E(I)nfection (concomitant outside biliary tree).

PORTAL HYPERTENSION

Causes

Extrahepatic:

(Blocked portal or splenic vein)	**I**nfection **I**nvasion (Tumor) **I**njury **I**atrogenic (biliary surgery) **I**diopathic (thrombosis)

Intrahepatic:

Presinusoidal	**A**denopathy (Lymphoma) **B**ilharziasis **C**irrhosis (biliary) **D**eposits (in liver in leukemia) **E(I)**diopathic **F**ibrosis (myelo)

Parenchymal

Cirrhosis **C**hiari (Budd-Chiari) syndrome **C**ystic liver disease **C**arcinoma	**C**ytotoxic drugs **C**lotting (Veno-occlusive disease) **C(S)**arcoid

Complications

Ascites
Bleeding (variceal)
Congestive gastropathy
Dynamic (hyper) circulation
Encephalopathy (Portosystemic)
Failure (Kidney).

HEPATOMEGALY

Causes

Apparent: Riedel's lobe, low diaphragm
Biliary obstruction (particularly extrahepatic)
Cirrhosis (early)
Decompensation: Congestive heart failure
E(I)nfection/Inflammation: Hepatitis. Abscess (amebic, pyemic). Schistosomiasis
Fatty liver
Growths and cysts: Ca, hydatid, polycystic
Hematological: Leukemia, lymphoma, myeloproliferative diseases
Hemochromatosis (or other metabolic diseases, e.g. amyloidosis, glycogen storage disease).

Enlarged Tender Liver

Abscess (amebic or pyogenic) or hepatitis (viral, alcoholic)
Budd-Chiari syndrome
CHF, Carcinoma of liver
Degeneration (or bleeding) into hepatoma.

HEPATOSPLENOMEGALY

Amyloidosis and storage disorders
Blood diseases: Chronic hemolytic anemia, pernicious anemia, leukemia, lymphomas
Constrictive pericarditis
Decompensation (cardiac)
E(I)nfection: Malaria, kala-azar, infective endocarditis, infective hepatitis, infectious mononucleosis.

GALLSTONES

Risk Factors

Cholesterol

Age: Elderly
Biliopancreatic bypass
Cystic fibrosis
Drugs: Octreotide, ceftriaxone
Endocrine: DM, pregnancy, sex hormones
Female sex. Fat
GI motility reduction: Parenteral nutrition
Hormone replacement therapy (also pregnancy, oral contraceptives)

Pigment

Chronic hemolysis
Cirrhosis
Complete parenteral nutrition
Chronic biliary infection
Clonorchis sinensis (causes stones which may contain dead parasites)

Complication	*Symptoms*	*Signs*
Stone impaction in common bile duct	Biliary colic	Upper abdominal tenderness
Acute cholecystitis	Fever, abdominal pain, nausea, vomiting	Tenderness and muscle guarding in right upper quadrant Murphy's sign
Chronic cholecystitis	Repeated attacks of biliary colic Epigastric discomfort	Localized tenderness in right hypochondrium Murphy's sign
Acute pancreatitis	Epigastric pain/ tenderness Vomiting	Epigastric pain radiating to back Discoloration of flanks
Acute cholangitis	Upper abdominal pain, fever with rigors, jaundice (Charcot's triad)	Added presence of bacteremia (Reynold's pentad)

PANCREATITIS

Acute Pancreatitis

Causes

Alcohol abuse
Biliary tract calculi
Cryptogenic
Drugs, e.g. thiazides, tetracyclines, valproate
Endocrine: Cushing's syndrome
Familial
Growths (Pancreatic)
Hypertriglyceridemia (types I and V)
Hypercalcemia
Hypothermia
Infections:
1. Viral: Mumps, Coxsackie-B, ECHO, Hepatitis A, B.
2. Bacterial: *Mycoplasma pneumoniae*

Injury: Blunt, penetrating, iatrogenic (ERCP, cardio-pulmonary bypass), scorpion bite.

Clinical Features

Abdominal pain (usually epigastric with tenderness)
Back radiation of pain
Confusion (due to hypoxia)
Dehydration
Emesis

Grey Turner's (and Cullen's) sign
Hypovolemic shock
Icterus (10–20%).

Diagnosis

Raised serum amylase: 3–4 times normal.
Peritoneal lavage: Amylase rich fluid.

Chronic Pancreatitis

Types

Alcoholic
Tropical (calcifying).

Causes

Chronic alcohol consumption
Cholelithiasis
Cystic fibrosis
Closure (obstruction) of sphincter of Oddi
Cirrhosis primary biliary.

Clinical Features

Pain

- Upper abdominal, pptd. by alcohol, heavy diet
- Relieved by jack-knife posture
- Backache

Pancreatic failure: Anorexia, steatorrhea, weight loss.
Pyrexia: Low grade.

Differential Diagnosis

	Alcoholic	*PCP*
Sex	Males	Females
Diabetes	Uncommon	Common
Steatorrhea	Common	Less frequent
Intraductal calculi	Uncommon	Frequent
Pancreatic cancer	Less likely	More likely

CHAPTER

2

Cardiovascular System

DYSPNEA

Physiological

Exercise, high altitude.

Pathological

Alveolar (Pulmonary): COPD, embolism
Blood disease: Anemia
Cardiovascular: IHD, cardiac failure
Diabetic acidosis (Also kidney failure)
Endocrine: Thyrotoxicosis
Fat (Obesity)
Gas (and other causes of abdominal distension)
Hysterical.

Paroxysmal Dyspnea

Low	Laryngeal: Foreign body, laryngismus stridulus
Cardiac	Cardiac: Acute LV failure, valvular disease, cardiac tamponade
Reserve	Respiratory: Bronchial asthma, spontaneous pneumothorax, acute pulmonary edema, pulmonary embolism.

Nocturnal Dyspnea

Cardiac: LVF, hypertrophic cardiomyopathy, coronary spasm
Pulmonary: Asthma, extrinsic allergic alveolitis, emboli
CNS/pharyngeal: Sleep apnea.

ACUTE CHEST PAIN

Acute coronary syndrome
Aortic dissection
Arrhythmia at onset
Colic (esophageal)
Cholecystitis (acute)
Pericarditis
Pulmonary embolism
Peptic ulceration
Pneumothorax (spontaneous)
Pneumonia.

Complications of AMI

1. Mechanical
2. Arrhythmias
3. Ischemic
4. Inflammatory
5. Embolic.

SYNCOPE

Causes: 3Cs

1. **Common faint** (vasovagal attack): Emotion, heat, carotid sinus hypersensitivity
2. **Cardiac:**
   a. Inadequate LV output: Arrhythmias, AS
   b. Inadequate LV filling: IHD, postural hypotension, cough, micturition, PPH
3. **Cerebral:** Hypoxia due to anemia.
   High altitude.
   Hypoglycemia.

RAISED JVP

Anemia
Bradycardia (marked)
Congestive heart failure
Decreased compliance (volume capacity) of RV—Pericardial effusion, constrictive pericarditis
Elevated intrathoracic pressure

Pressure on SVC
Pleural effusion (massive)
Fluid overload (IV)
Growths (or obstructive lesions) in right heart:
Tumor or thrombus in RA
TR or TS
Hyperdynamic states (besides Anemia):
Alcohol
Beriberi
Cor pulmonale (anoxic)
Diseases of liver
Exercise
Fever
Grave's disease
Heat
Pregnancy
Paget's disease.

CYANOSIS

Decreased Hb >5 g/100 mL blood (30% of total Hb in capillaries)
Deficient oxygenation of blood in lungs, e.g. pneumonia, chronic bronchitis
Decreased O_2 transfer across alveolar-capillary membrane, e.g. fibrosing alveolitis
Decreased amount of air ventilating the lungs, e.g. poliomyelitis.

Causes

A. **Central** (Skin, mucous membrane, limbs warm, clubbing)
   1. *Cardiac:* Cong. HD, Eisenmenger's, CHF (severe)
   2. *Respiratory:* COPD
   3. *High altitude:* Decreased O_2
   4. *Primary polycythemia:* Absolute excess of desaturated Hb.

B. **Peripheral:** (Skin only, limbs cold, no clubbing)
   Cold
   Cardiac failure
   Collapse (shock)
   Constriction (local).

Differential Cyanosis

Lower limbs only: Eisenmenger, PDA or interrupted aortic arch

Upper limbs only: Transposition of great arteries (TGA)

Left upper limb and both lower limbs: PDA with reversal of shunt in combination with pre-ductal coarctation of aorta

Intermittent: Ebstein's anomaly.

HEART SOUNDS

1st Heart Sound

Accentuated	Decreased	Variable	Split
MS, TS	MR, AS	CHB	Electrical delay
Tachycardia	Bradycardia	AF	RBBB
Short PR	Long PR	AFl	VPCs (LV)
WPW syndrome	LBBB	Changing block	Mechanical delay
AF, AFi	Myocarditis		Ebstein's
LA myxoma	Shock	Ectopics	MS
Floppy valve		VPT	LA myxoma
		Wenckebach	

2nd Heart Sound

			Split	
Accentuated	Decreased	Wide	Fixed	Paradoxical
A_2		RV abn:	ASD	Elec. LV
Hypertension	AS, AR, LVF	RBBB	RV	delay:
Aortic dil.		ASD	disease	LBBB
Exercise		APVD	VSD	WPW
AR (some)		PS	(large)	RV pacing
P_2		RVF		PVC (RV)
Mitral dis.,	PS	LV pacing		Mech. delay:
Pul. hyper.		PVCs (LV)		

Contd...

Contd...

Accentuated	Decreased	Wide	Split	
			Fixed	Paradoxical
LVF				AS, PDA
ASD		LV abn:		Myocardial
		VSD		disease
		MR		AR (severe)

3rd Heart Sound

Before 40: Physiological or pathological by the company it keeps.
After 40: To be considered pathological.

Left sided:
Hypertension
Myo. infarction
Cardiomyopathy

Right sided:
Massive pul. embolism
Cardiomyopathy

4th Heart Sound (Atrial Gallop)

Causes

High end-diastolic pressure–Early stage of Rt. or Lt. ventricular failure
Hypertrophy (severe ventricular), e.g. AS
(Atrial contraction has to produce considerable pressure rise to augment ventricular filling).

CARDIAC MURMURS

A. **Innocent:**

Systolic ejection
Soft
Short
Supine position best for auscultation
Supraclavicular or sternal border (Still's)
Single S_2 during expiration while standing
Satisfactory ECG and CXR.

B. **Physiological:**

Hyperkinetic:

Pregnancy
Pyrexia
Pulse pressure wide

Benign:

Pectus excavatum (severe)
Straight back syn.

C. **Relative:**

1. *Dilatational:* All 4 valve sites
2. *Flow:*

Mitral—VSD, PDA, MR Tri.—ASD, TR	Diastolic
Aortic—AR, aneurysm Pul.—Hemic, idiopathic dil. of artery	Systolic

D. **Organic:**

1. *Systolic:*

   a. Ejection:

Obstructive	Aortic/Pulmonary Supravalvar Valvar Infravalvar
Increased flow	AR Complete heart block
Postvalvar	Systemic hypertension Pulmonary hypertension 50/50 murmur (Atherosclerotic)

   b. Pansystolic:
   A-V valve incompetence—MR, TR
   L → R shunt—VSD, PDA

   c. Late systolic: Coarctation
   HOCM
   Mitral chorda or papillary muscle abnormality

2. *Diastolic:*

a. Obstruction at valves	MS, TS. Mid or late
b. Regurgitation across semilunar valves	AR, PR. Early
c. Increased flow across A-V valves	(Ref. functional murmurs)

3. *Continuous:*

a. Innocent:	Venous hum Mammary souffle Uterine souffle
b. Pathological:	5 pairs PDA, Aorto-pul. septal defect Pul. atresia, Fallot's tetral. Pul. AV fistula, systemic AV fistula Pul. arterial stenosis, coarctation Rupture of sinus of Valsalva into RA or RV, rupture of aortic aneurysm into rt. heart or pul. artery.

Mid-diastolic murmur: GAP

Graham Steel murmur
AR (mild)
PR (mild)

Beck's triad: 3 Ds

Decreased arterial pressure
Distended neck veins
Distant muffled heart sounds.

THE PULSE

Types of Abnormal: ABCDJPs

Alternans: LV failure
Anacrotic: AS
Bounding: Hyperkinetic states
Bisferiens: AR (severe) with moderate AS, HOCM
Corrigan:
  Physiological: Heat, pregnancy, alcohol
  Hyperkinetic states: e.g. thyrotoxicosis
  Cardiac: AR, PDA, VSD (large), complete heart block.
Dicrotic: Fevers (typhoid), severe CHF (usually secondary to dilated cardiomyopathy), tamponade, low output following aortic valve replacement for AR
Jerky: HOCM
Plateau: AS
Parvus et tardus: AS
Paradoxical: Pericardial effusion, constrictive pericarditis
  Pulmonary asthma.

Absent Pulse

Aortitis
Block (Atherosclerotic obstruction)
Coarctation
Dissection of aorta
Embolism
E(I)njury

CARDIAC ARRHYTHMIAS

Symptoms (Common to Many Arrhythmias)

1. **Local:** Palpitation, chest discomfort
2. **Reflex nervous:** Anxiety, sweating
3. **Cardiac:** Dyspnea, cardiac failure (occasional)

   Sinus bradycardia

   Rate <60/min. Non-cardiac or cardiac

   Sinus tachycardia

   Rate >100/min. Non-cardiac or cardiac

   Sinus arrhythmia

   Rate > with inspiration

   Premature (Ectopic) beats

   (Atrial, nodal, ventricular).

Causes

1. **Physiological:** Pregnancy.
2. **Pathological:**

   Ischemic heart disease

   Iatrogenic, e.g. digitalis

   Intoxicants: Excessive tea, coffee, tobacco, alcohol

   Irritation (Reflex), e.g. biliary or renal colic.

Diagnosis

1. Quick beat followed by long pause
2. Pulse apex deficit (<10/minute)
3. Abolished by exercise.

Malignant Premature Beats

>5/min	Multifocal
In pairs	R on T.

ATRIAL FIBRILLATION

Causes: THRILL

Thyrotoxicosis
Hypertensive heart disease
Rheumatic heart disease (MS)
Ischemic heart disease
Lung disease
Lone.

Types: 3Ps

Paroxysmal
Persistent
Permanent.

Diagnosis

1. Irregularly irregular, more after exercise
2. Pulse apex deficit (>10)
3. Changing 1st sound
4. Presystolic accentuation in MS disappears.

ATRIAL FLUTTER

Causes

Same as AF.

Diagnosis

1. Regular at 150/min
2. 'a' waves > radial pulse
3. Carotid sinus pressure slows rate.

PAROXYSMAL TACHYCARDIA

Supraventricular

Causes

Idiopathic (majority)
Ischemic heart disease
Iatrogenic: Digitalis
Inherited: WPW, LGL syndrome.

Diagnosis

1. Sudden onset and cessation
2. Rate >160/min
3. Carotid sinus slows supra, or restores sinus rhythm.

Treatment

Autonomic maneuvers
Break in pathway: Catheter or surgery
Cardioversion
Drugs: Adenosine, verapamil
E(I)mplantation devices.

Ventricular

Causes

IHD (majority).

Treatment

Cardioversion/defibrillation.

HEART BLOCK

S-A: Dropped beat (Whole PQRST drops out)

A-V: 1° Prolonged PR. Soft 1st sound

2° *Mobitz type I:* (Wenckebach) PR increases progressively till QRST is dropped

Mobitz type II:

Intermittent: Regular rhythm with sudden pauses.

Fixed: 2:1, 3:1, or 4:1. Regular 'a' waves 2, or 3 or 4 times >pulse rate

3° Complete.

Causes of Complete Heart Block

1. Congenital
2. Acquired: All Is

   Infarction

   Infection (rheumatic, diphtheria, syph.)

   Immunological (rheumatoid arth.)

   Infiltration (calcific AS, tumor, abscess)

   Iatrogenic (digitalis, cardiac surgery)

   Injury

   Irradiation.

Diagnosis: 4 Cs

Constant (rate) at 30–50/min.
Cannon waves
Cannon sounds
Corrigan pulse.

STOKES-ADAMS ATTACKS

If Heart Stops:
5 sec.: Giddiness
10 sec.: Unconsciousness
15 sec.: Convulsions

Causes:
Sick sinus syn.
Severe A-V block
Sinus (carotid) hypersensitivity
Subclavian steal syn.
Serious (malignant) VT.

SICK SINUS SYNDROME

Sinus bradycardia
Slow atrial fibrillation
Slow and fast rhythm (Brady-Tachy syndrome)
Sensitivity to beta-blocker
Junctional escape rhythm.

TACHYCARDIA

Regular

Sinus tachycardia
Supraventricular tachycardia
Ventricular tachycardia
Atrial flutter with 2:1 block.

Irregular

Atrial arrhythmias:
Fibrillation
Flutter with changing block
Tachycardia with block

Block: S-A or A-V with irregularly dropped beats
C(**S**)inus arrhythmia
Dissociation (A-V) with interference
Ectopic beats.

ECG Features of VT

Abnormal wide complexes (>0.14 sec.)
Bundle branch block (Rt. morphology)
Chest lead concordance
Deviation of axis (extreme)
Capture (fusion) beats.

BRADYCARDIA

1. **Sinoatrial dysfunction**
   Sinus bradycardia
   Sinus pauses: Sinus arrest
   Sinoatrial block 2:1 or >
2. **Atrioventricular block**
   Complete
   Partial 2:1 or >

COMMON VALVULAR DISEASES

	MS	MR	AR	AS
Common causes	Rheum. fever	Rheum. IE Ruptured papilla or chorda	Rheum. IE Syph. Cong.	Cong. Calcific Rheum.
Symptoms	Dyspnea Bronchitis Hemoptysis	Dyspnea	Dizziness Palpitation Dyspnea Angina	Angina Dyspnea Syncope Dizziness
Signs	Loud S_1 OS Mid-dias. murmur with presystolic accent	Pansystolic murmur Soft 1st 3rd sound at apex	Early dias. murmur LVH Peripheral signs	*Valvar:* Systolic thrill, murmur A_2 soft Ejection click *Supravalvar:* BP > rt. side No click. *Subvalvar* AR murmur No click

Complications (Common to all Valvular Diseases)

1. **A**rrhythmias
2. **B**acterial (infective) endocarditis
3. **C**ardiac failure

Also from compression in MR, MS: Hoarseness, dysphagia, collapse lung.

Mechanism of Hemoptysis in MS

Apoplexy (Rupture of pul. capillaries)
Bronchial veins rupture
Congestion (pulmonary)
Dema (edema)
Embolism (pulmonary).

MITRAL VALVE PROLAPSE

Clinical Features

Asymptomatic (or chest pain, palpitation, fatigue)
Bifid apical impulse
Click midsystolic (with or without late systolic murmur)
Death (sudden)
Echocardiography confirms diagnosis
Following conditions may be associated–IHD, ASD, HCM, Marfan's syn., WPW syn.
Gender : More in females.

CONGENITAL HEART DISEASE

Cyanosis at Birth: 2 As, 5 Ts

Atresia of aorta
Atresia of pulmonary artery
Tricuspid atresia

	ASD	PS	PDA	VSD	Coarctation
Ass. anomalies	APVD	VSD ASD Aortic root ano.	Isolated (usually)	PS	PDA bicuspid aort. valve Aneu. of sinus of Valsalva. Circle of Willis aneu. Ductus (also VSD)
Signs	Sys. mur. S_2 wide split	Mild harsh sys. mur. thrill, click P_2 delay Severe No click P_2 absent	Cont. machinery mur. Diff. cyanosis	Pansys. mur., thrill (4th LIS)	Delayed femorals Reversed Hill's Suzman's Ejection click Sys. mur
ECG	RBBB	RVH plus strain	LVH	LVH or LVH plus RVH	LVH
Radiology	Hilar dance	Oligemia Post- sten. dil.	Prominent pul. conus	Vascularity plus RVH	Rib notching Reversed 3 sign
Other features	Only cong. lesion in which acquired lesion may be present	Moon face (at times)	Compen. channel in Tetralogy Tricuspid atresia Transp.	Loudness and length of murmur inversely prop. to size of defect	4–5 times more in males Lower limbs less developed

Truncus arteriosus
Transposition of vessels
Tetralogy of Fallot
Total anomalous pul. venous drainage.

Common Lesions (if Child Survives Infancy)

Non-cyanotic:	RVH: ASD, PS
	LVH: PDA, VSD, Coarctation.
Cyanotic:	Tetralogy of Fallot

Single Gene Defects and Congenital Heart Disease

Noonan's syn.	Hypertrophic cardiomyopathy
	PS
	ASD
Marfan's syn.	Aortic root dilatation
	MVP
Holt-Oram syn.	ASD
	VSD (occasional)

Down's syndrome
40% have cong. heart disease
40% of these are A-V septal defects
Other lesions:

VSDs	30%
ASDs	10%
Fallot's	5%
PDA	5%.

Trilogy of Fallot: PS with reversed interatrial shunt.
Pentalogy of Fallot: Tetralogy + ASD.

Tetralogy

PS Overriding aorta
RVH VSD

1. Quiet cardiac impulse
2. Systolic thrill, murmur (due to PS)
3. S_2 loud and single.

X-ray: Couer en sabot, oligemia.

Transposition of the Great Arteries

1. Harsh sys. mur. left sternal border
2. S_2 +
3. 'Egg on string' appearance on X-ray.

Truncus (High VSD Associated)

1. Sys. thrill, murmur at base
2. S_2 loud and single
3. Cardiomegaly gross with wide supracardiac shadow.

Tricuspid Atresia (ASD or Patent Foramen Ovale)

1. Central cyanosis
2. Forceful apex impulse (LVH)
3. S_2 single (No P_2)
4. X-ray: Enlarged LV+RA; absent pul. conus.

Total Anomalous Pulmonary Venous Connection (TAPVC)

1. Signs like ASD (Continuous mur. in 25%)
2. X-ray: Figure of 8 (Snowman appearance).

Eisenmenger's Syndrome

1. Cyanosis: Uniform with VSD, may be differential with ductus
2. Dyspnea, syncope, angina, squatting (not common with PDA)
3. Palpable pulmonary pulsation, RV heave
4. P_2 accentuated
5. Graham Steell murmur
6. CXR: Dilatation of pulmonary trunk. Decreased peripheral vascular markings.

Note: VSD is associated with greatest shunt reversal, ASD moderate, PDA least.

Ebstein's Anomaly

- Central cyanosis may occur
- Triple rhythm
- Loud pansystolic murmur lower end of sternum due to TR
- Sudden attacks of PT
- CXR: Gross cardiomegaly, sharp (stencilled) outline of heart. Decreased vascularity of lung fields.

INFECTIVE ENDOCARDITIS

Predisposing Causes

Congenital:

Aneurysm of sinus of Valsalva
Bicuspid aortic valve
Coarctation of aorta
Ductus arteriosus
E(Vee) VSD

Acquired:

Most susceptible:
Mild MR or AR,
small VSD
Low risk:
ASD
Severe MS
Atrial fibrillation

Main organisms	Common sources of infection		Clinical features
Bacterial			
Str. viridans	Tooth extraction	Signs of infection	Fever Clubbing Spleen +
Staph. epidermidis	Genitourinary and rectal procedures	Ss. of heart disease	Cardiac lesion changing murmurs
Entero. faecalis	Cardiac surgery	Signs of embolism	Splinter hemorrhages Janeway lesions Hematuria
HACKE *Non-bacterial* Fungal Ricketssial		Immuno-logical phenomena	Osler's nodes Roth's spots Chro. nephritis

Surgical measures

Indications

Abscess formation
Biotic resistant organisms, e.g. *Coxiella*
Cardiac failure (acute or chronic due to valve destruction)
Drug addicts: Infected tricuspid valve
Early prosthetic valve endocarditis
Fungal infection.

Modes of Death

1. CHF
2. Mycotic aneurysm
3. Kidney failure.

ISCHEMIC HEART DISEASE

Risk Factors

Anxiety (Type A personality)
Body build
Cigarette smoking
Diabetes
Exercise lack
Family history
Gender—More in males
Hypertension
Hyperlipidemia
Hyperhomocysteinemia

Husband (incidence less in spinsters than married women).

ACUTE CORONARY SYNDROME

- Unstable angina (UA)
- Non-ST elevated MI (NSTEMI)
- ST elevated MI (STEMI).

Stable Angina Pectoris

Precipitating Factors: 7 Es

Exertion
Exercise (effort)
Emotion
Exciting programs on TV
Extramarital (or casual) sexual intercourse.
Extremes of temp. (cold)
Eating (large meal)

Clinical Features

Pain
Sudden onset
Short duration (seconds)
Substernal
Squeezing
Stopping or sublingual nitroglycerin or spray relieves.

Variant Angina (Prinzmetal's)

Pain of cyclic pattern, often at rest
Arrhythmias common
ST elevation (instead of depression).

Unstable Angina

Anginal pain at rest (>20 min)
Angina of recent onset, severe
Angina of effort with increasing frequency and duration
Angina destabilization (recent, crescendo)
Angina post MI.

Note: Angina with syncope more common in the elderly points to severe CAD.

Drug Therapy for Angina

Aspirin
ACE inhibitors
Antianginal drugs.

Complications of Acute MI

Early

Arrhythmias
Burst (Rupture): Vent. septal, cardiac
Collapse (Shock)
Dysfunction of papillary muscle
Embolism
Failure: LV or congestive.

Late

ASD
Aneurysm (ventricular)
Shoulder hand syndrome
Dressler's syndrome.

Myocardial Infarction due to Coronary Lesion other than Atheroma

Anomalous origin of coronary artery
Bulge (aneurysm) of coronary artery
Collagen disease: SLE, PAN
Dissecting aneurysm of cor. artery
Embolism (e.g. IE)
Fistula of cor. artery
Fibrosis following irradiation.

CARDIAC ARREST

Mechanism

Cardiac standstill (70%)
Ventricular fibrillation (30%).

Reversible Causes

Hypovolemia
Hypoxia
Hypothermia
Hypo or hyperkalemia
Hydrogen ions (acidosis).

Irreversible Causes

Tamponade
Thrombosis (MI, pulmonary embolism)
Tension pneumothorax
Trauma
Toxins.

SUDDEN CARDIAC DEATH

Causes

Arrhythmic RV dysplasia
Brugada syn.
Coronary heart dis. (most common)
Cong. or acquired Long QT syn.
Cardiomyopathies (hypertrophic or dilated).

Clinical Conditions

1. **Medical:**
   Apoplexy (cerebrovascular)
   Bleeding
   Cardiac infarction
   Drugs
   Drowning
   Embolism (acute pulmonary). Electric shock
2. **Surgery:** (including anesthesia)
3. **Diagnostic:** Cardiac catheterization, angio.

Diagnosis

Absent pulses
Breathing absent or gasping
Cyanosis
Coma
Dilated pupils.

Management

1. **Basic cardiac life support**
   Airway
   Breathing
   Circulation
2. **Advanced cardiac life support.**

HYPERTENSION

Causes

1. **Primary or Essential**
2. **Secondary**
   a. *Renal*
      Renal parenchymal
      Renovascular
   b. *Endocrinal*
      Cushing's syndrome
      Acromegaly
      Pheochromocytoma
      Primary aldosteronism
   c. *Vascular*
      Coarctation of aorta
      Nonspecific aortic arteritis
   d. *Drugs*
      Oral contraceptives
      Steroids
      NSAIDs
      Cyclosporin
   e. *Miscellaneous*
      Obstructive sleep apnea
      Thyroid disorder.

Treatment

1. **Non-pharmacological:** Lifestyle measures
   Alcohol
   Body weight
   Cigarette smoking
   Diet: Salt excess
   Exercise
2. **Pharmacological**
   ACE inhibitors
   α blockers
   β blockers
   α + β blockers
   CCBs
   Centrally acting drugs
   Diuretics
   Direct vasodilators.

Drug Interactions

Corticosteroids
Contraceptives
Carbenoxolone
Cyclosporin
Consumption of NSAIDs, tyrosine containing foods.

Malignant Hypertension: Triad of Rs

Raised diastolic pressure (>130 mm)
Retinopathy (including hemorrhages)
Renal damage (proteinuria, >blood urea).

Paradoxical Hypertension

Increase of BP in pts on anti-hypertensive therapy

1. β blockers in patients with DM and high BP
2. β blockers in patients with pheochromocytoma
3 Bilateral renal artery stenosis.

Hypertensive Crisis

Hypertensive Emergency

Malignant hypertension, e.g. BP >180/120
Abrupt drug withdrawal
Bad kidneys (e.g. Acute glomerulonephritis)
Catecholamine excess: Pheochromocytoma
Drugs: Steroids, sympathomimetics
Events involving CNS: CVA
Following coronary bypass surgery.

Treatment

Oral CCBs or ACEI/ARB.

Hypertensive Urgency (No End Organ Damage)

Accelerated hypertension
Brain infarct
C(S)urgical: Postoperative, after kidney transplant, severe body burns
Discontinuation (sudden) of antihypertensive therapy
Eclampsia.

Treatment

IV nitroglycerin, Enalaprilat or Labetalol.

HEART FAILURE

Acute Heart Failure

Causes

1. **LV myocardial dysfunction:**
   Ischemia and infarction.
   Infection: Myocarditis (and cardiomyopathy).
   Iatrogenic: Cardiac depressant drugs.
2. **Increased LV load:**
   Systolic (Pressure) overload: Hypertension, AS
   Diastolic (Volume) overload: MR, AR, VSD, PDA.
3. **Arrhythmias.**

Clinical Features

Alternans pulse
Basal crackles
Cold clammy skin
Dyspnea
Elevated JVP
Fast pulse
Gallop rhythm
Hypotension.

Treatment of Acute LV Failure

Decubitus: Propped up

Dopes: Inj. Diamorphine
Deliver O_2
Diuretics (IV)
Dopamine to increase cardiac output (if necessary)
Determine cause, e.g. myo. infarct
Diverse measures:
Intra-aortic balloon pump. Anti-arrhythmic therapy. Emergency cardioversion.

Chronic Congestive Heart Failure

Causes

1. **RV myocardial dysfunction (rare):** Myocarditis, cardiomyopathy
2. **Systolic overload of RV:** Preceding LVF (commonest cause), pulmonary hypertension, chronic cor pulmonale, PS
3. **Diastolic overload:** Left to right shunt, e.g. ASD
4. **Restriction of RV:** EMF, constrictive pericarditis (localized).

Symptoms

Due to Back Pressure

Cerebral: Headache, insomnia, sluggish mental state
Pulmonary: Cough, dyspnea
Portal: Anorexia, nausea, hepatic angina
Peripheral: Swelling of feet, face.

Signs

Elevated JVP
Enlarged, tender liver
Enlarged heart
Edema feet, anasarca.

Treatment

Decubitus: Rest in bed
Diet: Salt restricted, small feeds
Diuretics
Digitalis
Decreasing:
 Preload: Nitrates
 After load: Vasodilators. ACE inhibitors

Diverse measures: O_2, anticoagulants (to prevent venous thrombosis). Treatment of underlying cause, e.g. valvular heart disease, anemia, thyrotoxicosis.

Diastolic Heart Failure

- More in elderly especially those with long-standing hypertension or other hypertrophic ventricular disease
- Classical signs of heart failure but small heart
- Characteristic abnormalities of diastolic LV dysfunction on echo.

Refractory Heart Failure

Aneurysm (ventricular)
BP raised
Carditis
Dysrhythmia
Embolism (pulmonary)
Failure to take treatment
Gross anemia
Hidden (occult) heart disease: AS, MS.

COR PULMONALE

Acute Cor Pulmonale (Pulmonary Embolism)

Predisposing Factors

Pathological triad	Clinical triad
Blood stasis	Post-operative (or fracture)
Blood vessel wall trauma	Post-partum
Blood clotting abnormality (hypercoagulability)	Post-trauma (major)

Deep Vein Thrombosis (See later)

Presentation of Pulmonary Embolism

	Acute minor	Acute major	Chronic
Dyspnea	Mild	Severe	Chronic progressive

Chest pain	Pleuritic	Acute, dull central	Exertional, dull, central
Tachycardia	Mild	Usually marked	Variable
BP	Normal	Low	Normal until late
Cyanosis	No	Common	Common
Edema	No	Not acutely	Common
JVP	Normal	Raised	Raised
Heart sounds	Normal	S_3	S_3, S_4, P_2+
Chest X-ray	Often normal	Usually abnormal	Abnormal
ECG	Usually normal	Usually abnormal	Abnormal

Subacute Cor Pulmonale

1. **Asphyxial:** Bronchitis, asthma
2. **Malignant:** Miliary carcinomatosis of lung.

Chronic Cor Pulmonale

Causes

Parenchyma: Chronic bronchitis, emphysema, bronchiectasis, pneumoconiosis.

Cage (thoracic): Kyphoscoliosis, Pickwickian syn., thoracoplasty, myopathy, myasthenia

Vessels: Recurrent pul. embolism, PPH, PAN, sickle cell anemia.

Clinical Features

1. Compensated stage: Ss. of primary disease + RVH
2. Decompensated stage: Signs of RVF.

PULMONARY HYPERTENSION

Causes

1. **Idiopathic:** Practically confined to females.
2. **Secondary:** Hypertrophic pulmonary osteoarthropathy
3. **Hyperkinetic:** Increased pulmonary blood flow because of R-L shunt, e.g. VSD, ASD, PDA, truncus
4. **Passive:** LVF, MS, MR
5. **Obstructive:** Parenchymal lung disease, Embolic
6. **Active:**
   High altitude
   Hyperventilation.

Signs

Inspection: Peripheral cyanosis
Palpation: Pulse small
Parasternal heave
Auscultation:
Sounds: S_2 closely split, P_2+
RA and RV gallop
Ejection systolic click

Murmurs: Systolic ejection
Early diastolic
Pansystolic of relative TR.

Treatment

Bosentan
Sildenafil
Ambrisentan.

CARDIOVASCULAR SYPHILIS

Clinical Manifestations: 4As

1. **Aortitis**

Always	Aortalgia
Trust	Tambour A_2
Medical	Murmur (aortic systolic)
Colleague	Calcification of ascending aorta.

2. **Angina**
   Differs from angina of atheromatous origin thus:
   Longer duration
   Myocardial infarction rare but fatal
   Nitroglycerin less effective
   Often nocturnal.
3. **Aortic regurgitation**
   Angina more common
   Better audibility of mur. in 2nd RIS
   Calcification of ascending aorta
   Diastolic thrill common.
4. **Aneurysm.**

Ascending Arch (Aneurysm of Signs)

Signs: Pulsation in 2nd RIS
Systolic and early dias. mur.
Pulse, BP < on rt. side

Symptom: Bovine cough.

Transverse and Descending Arch (Aneurysm of Symptoms)

Clinical Features

Due to compression of:

Tubes	Trachea, bronchus—cough, dyspnea, Esophagus—dysphagia
Vessels	Veins—edema face, prominent veins Arteries—radial pulse, BP > in left arm
Nerves	Left recurrent laryngeal—hoarseness Cervical sympathetic—Horner's Vagus—tachycardia Phrenic—hiccough, left dome paralysis Intercostal, brachial plexus—chest or left arm pain
Bones	Deep seated pain from erosion.

AORTIC DISSECTION

Predisposing Causes

Atherosclerosis
BP high
Bicuspid aortic valve

Coarctation (Also cystic medial necrosis, Marfan's)
Dominance: Male
E (I)njury
Female: Third trimester of pregnancy
Giant cell arteritis
Hypertension.

Clinical Features: 5Ps

Pain: Severe, maximum at onset, radiation into lower half of body
Pericarditis
Peripheral pulses weak or absent
Peripheral failure (Shock)
Pyrexia: Low grade.

MIDDLE AORTIC SYNDROME

Takayasu's arteritis.

Clinical Features: 4Cs

Cardiovascular: Diminished or absent peripheral pulsations
Cerebrovascular: In carotid and vertebral artery territory
Claudication
Cutaneous changes: Ulceration of nose or lips, loss of hair.

HEART MUSCLE DISEASE

Heart muscle disease can be idiopathic, genetic or specific.

Cardiomyopathies

Classification

1. **Dilated:** Dilated hypokinetic LV in absence of valvular, coronary, hypertensive or systemic disease
   Enlargement of the cavity of the ventricle
   Modes of presentation: MALE
   MR: Murmur
   Arrhythmia: AF or ventricular
   LV failure
   Embolism: Pulmonary or systemic
   Echo: Dilated LV and global hypokinesia
   Special forms:
   Postpartum cardiomyopathy
   Arrhythmogenic RV cardiomyopathy
2. **Hypertrophic**
   Hypertrophy of undilated LV not due to pressure or volume overload

Symptoms	*Signs*
Angina	Jerky pulse
Syncope	Apex impulse double
Dyspnea	Murmur: Late ejection systolic

Echo: Abnormal wall thickening

3. **Restrictive**
   Stiff vent. which restricts filling
   TR and enlarged LA and RA
   Clinical Features
   Rt. sided: Like constrictive pericarditis
   Lt. sided: MR. Atrial fibrillation.

Specific Heart Muscle Disease

Etiology

Alcohol
Blood disease: Hemochromatosis (primary)
Congenital (and familial): Noonan's syn., Friedreich's ataxia
Drugs: Cytotoxic chemotherapy, lithium
Endocrine: Pheochromocytoma, thyrotoxicosis
Fibrosis: Endomyocardial
Growths: Malignant melanoma
Hypereosinophilic (Loeffler's) syndrome
Infiltration: Lymphoma, amyloid, sarcoid
Intestinal parasites in children.

Myocarditis

Causes: 5 Is

1. **I**mmune disorders: Rheumatic fever, rheumatoid arthritis, serum sickness
2. **I**nfection:
   Viral—Influenza, HIV, dengue, hepatitis E

Bacterial—Diphtheria, pneumonia
Rickettsial—Rocky mountain spotted fever, Q fever. Typhus
Spirochetal—Relapsing fever, Lyme carditis, syphilis.
Protozoal—Tryp. Cruzi, toxoplasmosis
Parasitic—Trichinosis, schistosomiasis, echinococcus.

3. **I**atrogenic: Phenothiazines, lithium, cocaine, quinidine, theophylline, cyclophosphamide.
4. **I**rradiation
5. **I**nsect bite: Wasp sting
6. **I**mmunological: SLE, scleroderma, PAN.

Signs: 3 Ts

- Tachycardia (disproportionate to signs of infection)
- Tachyarrhythmias
- Tic-tac rhythm.

PERICARDITIS

Causes: All Is

Idiopathic
Infections: Bacterial, viral (e.g. influenza, HIV, respiratory syncytial virus, mumps), fungal, parasitic, spirochetal
Immunological: Rheumatic fever, lupus erythematosus, RA

Infarction (myocardial)
Infiltration (malignant)
Insufficiency: Kidney (uremia), thyroid
Iatrogenic: Drug-induced, serum sickness
Injury: To chest
Irradiation.

Acute Pericarditis

Symptom: Pain
Sign: Friction rub
ECG: ST elevation with saddle back concavity.

Pericardial Effusion

Symptoms	**Signs**
Chest (precordial) distress	**D**ullness in 2nd LIS and outside apex beat
Compression symptoms	**D**iminished—
Constitutional symptoms	Heart sounds
	Cardiac pulsations
	Voltage of ECG.

Hemorrhagic Effusion

Infection: TB
Injury
Infarction (myocardial)
Infiltration: Malignancy
Insufficiency: Kidney (uremia)
Iatrogenic: Anticoagulants.

Cardiac Tamponade

Beck's Triad

1. Rising venous pressure
2. Falling arterial pressure
3. Small quiet heart.

Constrictive Pericarditis

Causes

Infection: TB (majority), pyogenic
Irradiation of chest
Injury: Following hemopericardium (Trauma, surgery)
Idiopathic: Acute benign pericarditis
Immunological: Collagen disease, e.g. rheumatoid arthritis.

Signs

Of constriction:	*Of pericardial involvement:*
JVP raised	Paradoxical pulse
Kussmaul's sign	Knock sound
Ascites	Calcification of pericardium.

SHOCK

Causes

Clean SHAVEN Doctor
Clean Cardiogenic (Myocardial infarction, arrhythmias)

Septicemic (Gram –ve septicemia)
Hypovolemic (Hemorrhage, gastroenteritis)
Anaphylactic (Drugs, bee or wasp sting)
Vascular (Pulmonary embolism, aortic dissection)
Endocrine (Acute adrenocortical insufficiency)
Neurogenic (Anesthesia, testicular trauma)
Doctor Drug-induced (Poisons, ganglion-blockers).

Clinical Features

Due to:

1. **Fall in cardiac output:** Pallor, hypotension, sweating, tachycardia, subnormal temp
2. **Inadequate perfusion of vital organs:**
   a. *Kidneys:* Oliguria
   b. *Brain:* First restlessness, later apathy; coma
   c. *Liver:* Metabolic acidosis
   d. *Heart:* Coronary insufficiency
3. **Shock lung.**

ORTHOSTATIC HYPOTENSION

Causes

Autonomic insufficiency (primary)
Bed rest (prolonged)
CNS disease: Syringo. tabes
Drugs: Vasodilators
Endocrine: Addison's, pheochromo, diabetes
Following sympathectomy

Guillain-Barre syndrome
Hyponatremia
Hypovolemia
Idiopathic.

PERIPHERAL VASCULAR DISEASE

Symptoms: 6 Ps

Pain	**P**aralysis
Pallor	**P**ulselessness
Paresthesia	**P**erishing with cold

Advice: Stop smoking, start walking.

Gangrene

Causes: RESTED

Raynaud's
Ergot (and other drugs)
Senility
Thrombosis
Embolism
Diabetes

Arterial Thrombosis

Risk Factors

Antiphospholipid antibody syn.
Blood disease: Polycythemia

Cigarette smoking
Diabetes mellitus
Ergot
Family history
Gender: Male
Hypertension
Hyperfibrinogenemia
Hyperlipidemia
Hyperhomocysteinemia
Increased factors VII and VIII.

Deep Vein Venous Thrombosis (DVT)

Antiphospholipid antibody syn.
Blood disease: Myeloproliferative disorders
CHF
Dehydration
E(I)nactivity (post-operative)
Fat (obesity)
Growths (Malignant)
Hyperviscosity syn.
Hormone treatment
Inflammatory bowel disease
Journey (long air)
Kidney disease (Nephrosis)
Varicose veins, pregnancy.

Diagnosis of DVT

- **D**-dimer (>50 ng/mL) in 50%
- **D**oppler ultrasonography.

INTERMITTENT CLAUDICATION

Differential Diagnosis

Type	Pain relief	Pain site	Signs	Tests
Arterial	Standing still	Calf	Absent distal pulses	Ankle: arm systolic ratio <0.8
Neuro-logical	Lying down 1/2 hr	Along derma-tome	Abnormal after exercise of chronic	MRI
Venous	Leg elevation	Calf	Venous insufficiency	Venogram
Rheo-logical	Standing still	Whole leg	Bounding pulses	Full blood count, ESR

Clues to Renal Artery Stenosis

- Atherosclerosis (known)
- Age: Onset of hypertension before 30 or after 55 years
- Adverse rise in previously controlled high BP
- Abnormality of kidneys (Discrepancy of kidney size)

- **Accelerated or resistant hypertension**
- **Abdominal bruit**
- **Azotemia not otherwise explained or worsened, ACE inhibitors or Angiotensin II receptor blockers**
- **Abrupt onset of pulmonary edema (or recurrent CHF) in hypertensive patient, particularly with preserved LV function.**

CHAPTER 3

Respiratory System

COUGH

Causes

1. **In resp. tract:**
   Pharyngeal (and Laryngeal): Infection
   Pulmonary: Pneumonia, TB
   Pleural effusion, bronchiectasis
   Pneumothorax
   Pressure: Mediastinal growth, aneurysm
2. **Outside resp. tract:**
   Auditory: Wax or inflammation
   Abscess: Liver, subphrenic
   Anxiety.

Types

Asthmatic: Mostly nocturnal
Bovine: Vocal cord paralysis
Croupy: Laryngeal infection
Dry: TB
Expectorant: Bronchitis, bronchiectasis

Fetid: Anaerobic infection
Gander (metallic): Mediastinal compression
Hacking: Postnasal drip
Intermittent (Staccato): Whooping cough.

Nocturnal

Asthma: Bronchial, cardiac (LVF)
Angiotensin converting enzyme inhibitor
Aspiration: Post-nasal drip, GER.

HEMOPTYSIS

Causes

1. **Pulmonary**
   Infection: TB, bronchiectasis, lung abscess, aspergilloma
   Infiltration: Carcinoma, adenoma
   Infarction
   Injury: Contusion, transbronchial biopsy
   Immunological: SLE, polyarteritis, Goodpasture's syn.
   Idiopathic: Primary pul. hypertension
   Infection: Lung fluke
   Inherited: Hereditary hemorrhagic telangiectasia.
2. **Cardiovascular:** MS
3. **Bleeding diathesis:** Thrombocytopenia (severe), anticoagulants.

CLUBBING

1. **Pulmonary:**
   Abscess, **A**sbestosis
   Bronchiectasis
   Carcinoma bronchus
   Diffuse fibrosing alveolitis
   Empyema (chronic)
   Fibrosis (cystic)
2. **Cardiac:**
   Cyanotic cong. heart disease
   Infective endocarditis
3. **Extrathoracic:**
   Endocrine: Thyroid acropachy
   Familial or idiopathic
   Gastrointestinal disease: Crohn's disease
   Hepatic disease: Cirrhosis.

FOUL SMELLING SPUTUM

Abscess
Bronchiectasis
Carcinoma (breaking down)
Diaphragmatic abscess (bursting into lung)
Empyema (bursting into lung)
Fetid bronchitis
Gangrene lung.

RESPIRATORY SIGNS

Hyper-resonant Note

Air in pleural cavity
Bulla
Cavity
Cyst
Distension of stomach
Diaphragmatic eventration
Diaphragmatic hernia
Emphysema.

Impaired or Dull Note

Abscess
Bronchogenic Ca
Collapse, **C**onsolidation
Diaphragm raised (uncommon)
Effusion (and thickened pleura)
Fibrosis of lung.

Bronchial Breath Sounds

Types	**Causes**
Cavernous	Consolidation
Amphoric	Cavity
Tubular	Collapse.

Vocal Resonance

Increased: Consolidation
Cavity (superficial)

Decreased: Air in pleural cavity
Bronchial obstruction
Collapse
Diaphragmatic hernia
Effusion, emphysema
Fibrosis.

Crackles (Rales)

Abscess, ARDS
Bronchiectasis
Consolidation
Decompensation (Cardiac)
Edema
Fibrosis.

Wheezes (Rhonchi)

Polyphonic	**Monophonic**
More expiratory	Insp. or expiratory
Large number	Single or few
Not widely heard	Wide conduction
Loud. Can be heard with unaided ear	Cannot be heard with unaided ear (except stridor).

Causes

Congestion or thickening of mucus lining
Constriction of smooth ms. of bronchi
Chronic bronchitis, emphysema.

If single wheeze on inspiration—Stenosis or FB or lymph node or Ca obstructing principal bronchus.

Pleural Rub

Audible during both phases of respiration
Better heard on increased pressure of stethoscope
Cough does not change rub
Defined area (Localized)
Eliminated by holding breath
Frequently associated with localized pain and tenderness
Grating in character.

Succussion Splash

Hydropneumothorax
Herniation of stomach or colon into thorax
Huge cavity with fluid and air.

LUNG FUNCTION TESTS

A. **Airway function:** By spirometry

Test	Normal values	Comment
PEF (Peak exp. flow)	Wide normal range 300–700 L/min	Reduced in: Narrowing of airways Neuromuscular causes Useful for monitoring changes in bron. asthma
VC (Vital capacity)	3–6 L	Reduced in both restrictive and obstructive disorders
FVC (Forced vital capacity)	As for VC	As for VC
FEV_1 (Forced expir. vol. in 1 sec.)	75–80% of normal VC	Useful indicator of severity of obstructive disease
FEV_1/VC ratio	>70%/in males <75% in females	<70% diagnostic of airflow obstr. (except when VC is high) >85% in lung fibrosis

FEV_1 can be expressed thus

1. Volume-time curve: In pulmonary emphysema with reduced elastic recoil and very collapsible airways, FEV_1 is low even when airways are patent.
2. Flow-volume curve: In healthy individuals, maximal expiratory flow rate decreases steadily throughout forced expiration. This representation of maximal flow is useful for demonstrating:
   a. Reduction during middle of forced expiration is caused by small airways diseases (even when FEV_1 and FVC are normal)
   b. In emphysema, peak flow is well preserved but flow rates diminish early in expiration
   c. In obstruction of airway outside the thorax, flow is constant through first part of expiratiration rather than decelerating.

B. **Lung volumes:**

Total lung capacity (TLC): Volume of air in lungs after maximal inspiration (70%). Remaining 30% residual volume (RV) measured by spirometry, gas dilution and plethysmography

All lung volumes decreased—Parenchymal disease.

Increased RV-Airway disease

Increased TLC—Loss of elastic recoil, e.g. emphysema, cysts, bullae

Raised TLC and VC—Weak respiratory muscles.

C. **Carbon monoxide gas transfer factor:**
(Diffusing capacity).
Reduced
1. Reduction of alveolar capillaries:
   Emphysema
   Embolic diseases
   Endarteritis
   Fibrosis
2. Increased ventilatory perfusion mismatch:
   Pneumonia
   Pulmonary infections and infiltrations
3. Reduced Hb
4. Heavy smokers (High level of carboxy Hb).

Increased
1. Asthma
2. Alveolar hemorrhage
3. Polycythemia.

D. **Arterial blood gas values:**
Respiratory failure: PaO_2 <8 kPa (with or without CO_2 retention).
Ventilatory failure: $PaCO_2$ >7 kPa and PO_2 <8 kPa.

Causes of Inadequate Oxygenation: AIDS

Altitudes (High)
Impaired gas exchange
Diminished ventilation
Shunts.

BRONCHIECTASIS

Causes

Congenital

Cysts (bronchial)

Cystic fibrosis

Ciliary dyskinesia syn. (Kartagener's syn, immobile cells)

Ciliary (Mucociliary clearance deficiency)

Complement deficiency

Chronic granulomatous dis. (primary immune deficiency). Also hypogammaglobulinemia.

Acquired

Children:

Necrotizing pneumonia (Measles, whooping cough, staphylococcal, influenza, adenovirus)

Primary TB

Inhalation of foreign body.

Adults:

Allergic bronchopulmonary aspergillosis

Bronchial obstruction

Pulmonary TB

Suppurative pneumonia

Post-lung transplantation.

Clinical Presentation

1. Bronchitis
2. Bronchiectasis sicca (Hemoptysis)
3. Bronchial obstruction (partial) with relatively rapid onset
4. Bullous (drumstick) appearance of fingernails (pulmonary osteoarthropathy).

PNEUMONIA

Clinical Classification

1. Community acquired (CAP)
2. Nosocomial (Hospital acquired)
3. Ventilation associated
4. Aspiration pneumonia
5. Acute pneumonia in immune compromised hosts.

Causes

Primary: 4 Is

Infection:

Bacterial: *Pneumococcus, Staphylococcus, Streptococcus*
Viral: Influenza, respiratory syncytial
Rickettsial: Typhus
Mycoplasmal: *M. pneumoniae*
Yeast and fungi: Candida, actinomyces, histoplasma
Protozoa and parasites: Toxoplasma, amoeba.

Immunological: Polyarteritis
Irritation: Gas: Chlorine, ammonia, SO_2
Liquids: Vomit, lipid pneumonia.
Irradiation.

Secondary

In association with:
Aspiration from nasopharynx
Bronchiectasis
Carcinoma of lung
Depression of defenses:
Systemic disease
Steroids
Suppressive (immuno) drugs.

Special Features

Pneumococcal:	Lobar consolidation. Can result in most severe pneumonia. Good resolution
Staphylococcus:	Abscess formation
H. influenzae:	Principally in patients with underlying chest disorder (e.g. COPD)
Legionella spp.:	Important cause of CAP and nosocomial pneumonia. Often severe illness
Klebsiella:	Blood tinged sputum. Patchy consolidation
Tuberculous:	Usually apical. No response to antibiotics

Viral: More symptoms than signs
Fungal: *Pneumocystis jirovecii* in AIDS.

Slow Resolution of Pneumonia

Antibiotic resistance
Bronchial obst., bronchiectasis
Complications: Abscess, empyema
Diagnostic error, e.g. pul. embolism, bronchial Ca, fibrosing alveolitis
Endocarditis and other metastatic complications.
Faulty (inadequate) dosage
General factors: Hypoxia, dehydration, immunocompromised.

Recurrent Pneumonia

1. **Respiratory disease:**
   a. *Bronchial obstruction—*
      Intraluminal: Foreign body
      Intramural: Growth, stenosis
      Extramural: Compression by lymph nodes
   b. *Local bronchopulmonary disease—*
      Localized bronchiectasis
      Carnified lung due to chronic pneumonia
   c. *Generalized—*
      Bronchiectasis, cystic fibrosis, chronic bronchitis.
2. **Non-respiratory disease:**
   a. *Recurrent aspiration:* Alcoholics, epileptics
   b. *Immune deficiency states.*

LUNG ABSCESS

Causes

Aspiration
Bronchial obstruction
Consolidation. Carcinoma
Diaphragmatic
Embolic
Fungal (and other necrotising) infections.

Signs:	**Treatment:**
Consolidation or	Chemotherapy
Cavitation	Drainage
Clubbing	Excision

CYSTIC FIBROSIS

Clinical Presentation

1. **Respiratory 40%:** Bronchiolitis, bronchitis, bronchiectasis, pneumonia, sinusitis.
2. **Non-respiratory:**
   Malabsorption 30%
   Meconium ileus 20%
3. **Miscellaneous 10%:** Cirrhosis, infertility, nasal polyps, pancreatic insufficiency.

Diagnosis

Sweat test: Sodium or chloride levels in sweat >65 mEq/liter.

Guthrie test: Immunoreactive trypsin levels increased 2–3 times.

Treatment

Recombinant human DNase nebulized od. Pancreatic enzymes.

BRONCHIAL ASTHMA

Allergic	**Non-allergic**
Inhaled: Pollen, dust, smoke, fumes	Worry
	Infection
Ingested: Eggs, fish, nuts, strawberries	Drugs (aspirin, β-blockers)
	Exercise

Extrinsic	**Intrinsic**
Allergic history (eczema)	No his. of allergy
Brief attacks	Persistent
Childhood	Adult
Dermal test +ve, drug response good	-ve dermal test, poor response to drugs
E(IgE) raised	Low IgE
Family history	No family history
Good prognosis	Poor prognosis

Factors Promoting Asthma

Allergens (including occupational exposure)
Beta-blockers (and aspirin)
Cold air or exertion

Day time (early morning or night)
Emotion (or stress).

Danger Signs in Acute Attacks

Absent breath sounds (Silent lung)
BP low
Cyanosis
Decreased ability to talk
Exhaustion
Failure to respond to normal medication
Gross over-inflation of lungs (X-ray)
Hypoxia (Arterial PO_2 <8 kPa)
Increased pulse rate (>130) and pulsus paradoxus.

Management of Chronic Asthma

Steps

1. Occasional use of relief bronchodilators
2. Regular inhaled anti-inflammatory agents
3. High or low dose inhaled corticosteroids, plus long-acting inhaled β-agonist
4. High dose inhaled corticosteroids and regular bronchodilators
5. Addition of regular corticosteroid tablets.

CHRONIC OBSTRUCTIVE PULMONARY DISEASE

Risk Factors for COPD

1. **Genes**
2. **Exposure to particles**
    - Tobacco smoke

- Indoor air pollution from heating and cooking with fuel in poorly ventilated homes
- Occupational dusts: Coal and gold, organic, inorganic
- Outdoor air pollution.

3. **Reduced lung volume**
   - Lung growth and development
   - Previous tuberculosis
   - Recurrent lower resp. tract infections in early childhood
   - Poor nutrition.

Clinical Picture in Severe COPD

Pink puffer	**Blue bloater**
Pink (normal color)	Cyanosed, CHF
Poorly built (thin)	Obese
Pursed lip breathing	Mild dyspnea
Poor sputum vol.	Large sputum vol.
Polycythemia rare	Polycythemia common
Persists to keep PCO_2 down	Gives up and settles for poor blood gases
Prognosis poor	Remissions.

Management

Aminophylline
Anticholinergics (e.g. ipratropium)
Acebrophylline

Bronchodilator therapy
Corticosteroids
Domiciliary oxygen therapy
End to smoking.

EMPHYSEMA

Anatomical Types

Centriacinar: Bronchioles, alveolar ducts and alveoli are destroyed. More extensive in upper lobes.
Panacinar: Entire acinus destroyed. More extensive in lower lobes.

Clinical Types

Generalized	*Localized*
Hypertrophic	Obstructive
Atrophic	Compensatory
	Interstitial

Hypertrophic Emphysema: Clinical Features

Accessory muscle of resp. active, angle of Louis prominent
Breath sound diminished
Barrel chest
Costal angle wide
Diaphragm depressed
Decreased distance between suprasternal notch and lower margin of cricoid

Elevated shoulders
Fossae (supraclavicular) flattened out or bulged
Generalized airway obstruction
Horizontal ribs
Inspiratory expansion position of chest.

PULMONARY TUBERCULOSIS

Risk Factors

Age: Any
Bad environment
Contact with smear positive patients
Drugs: Corticosteroids, cytotoxic drugs
Endocrine: Diabetes
Faulty habits: Alcoholism, drug addiction
Gross undernutrition
HIV infection
Industrial lung disease, e.g. silicosis.

Primary Infection

Ghon lesion (Subpleural pul. lesion + regional lymphadenopathy).

Result

Resolution (Calcification) or Spread

1. **H**ematogenous:
   Acute: Miliary TB
   Chronic: Kidneys, bones, joints, meninges

2. **Lung component:** Cavitation or pleural effusion.
3. **Lymph node:** Bronchial obstruction (collapse or consolidation).

Post-primary (Re-infection)

Presentations: A to I, 3Ps

Asymptomatic. **A**menorrhea in females
Bronchial asthma
Cough (persistent). **C**onsolidation
Dyspepsia. **D**ecrease in weight
Effusion
Fatigue
Geriatric or senile (bronchitis or emphysema)
Hemoptysis
Hoarseness of voice
Injury (following to chest)
Infectious disease (measles, whooping cough)
Pleurisy
Pneumonia
Pyrexia of unknown origin.

Result

1. Healing with fibrosis.
2. Rupture into bronchus (bronchopneumonia, pneumonia).
3. Hematogenous spread: Miliary TB.

MILIARY TUBERCULOSIS

Choroidal tubercles in fundus (pathognomonic)
Dyspnea (and cyanosis) out of proportion to chest signs
Elevated pulse rate
Fever
Gradual onset
Hepatosplenomegaly
Miliary mottling on chest X-ray.

COLLAPSE OF THE LUNG

Causes

1. **Bronchostenosis:**
   Bronchial obstruction
   a. *In lumen:* Foreign body, mucus plugs
   b. *In wall:* Tumor
   c. *Outside wall:* Aneurysm, lymph node, tumor
2. **Compression collapse:**
   Lymphadenopathy
   Pneumothorax, pleural effusion.

Signs

Dullness on percussion
Diminished: Movement, vocal resonance, breath sounds
Deviation of mediastinum (to same side).

LUNG CAVITY

Causes:

Pulmonary TB (commonest) +
Abscess
Aspergillosis
Bulla
Cyst: Congenital, hydatid
Carcinoma (breaking down)
Caplan's nodules
Degenerating tumor
Embolism (pul. infarction)
Fibrosis (progressive massive)
Granuloma (Wegener's).

Signs:

Cracked-pot resonance
Cavernous (or amphoric) breath sounds
Pectoriloquy
Post-tussive suction

LUNG FIBROSIS

1. **Localized**
   Infection: Pneumonia, abscess, TB
   Infarction
   Irradiation
2. **Diffuse interstitial**
   Alveolitis extrinsic allergic
   Breathing in dust (Pneumoconiosis)
   C(S)arcoidosis
   Drugs: NFT, busulphan, amiodarone
   E(I)rradiation

Fibrosing alveolitis
Growths: Carcinomatosis
Hypertension: Pulmonary venous
Interstitial lung dis.: Asbestosis
Immune disorders: SLE, systemic sclerosis.

Signs

Diminished movements, VR, breath sounds
Deviation of mediastinum (to same side)
Dull note.

OCCUPATIONAL AIRWAY DISEASE

Types of Lung Reactions

Asthma
Bronchitis, emphysema
Cancer of lung or pleura
Degenerative changes in lung parenchyma
Extrinsic allergic alveolitis
Fibrosis
Granulomatous reactions, e.g. berylliosis.

Clinical Features

Depend on type of inhalation:

1. **Acute tracheobronchitis:** Gases or metallic fumes
2. **Pneumoconioses:**
   Minerals: Asbestos, silica, coal, talc
   Metals: Aluminum, beryllium, iron ore.

BRONCHOGENIC CARCINOMA

Etiology

Atmospheric pollution
Bronchitis (chronic)
Cigarette smoking
Dominant sex (more in males)
Exposure (occupation, e.g. radioactive gases, asbestos)
Fibrosis of lung
Genetic factors.

Cell Types

A(E)pidermoid	Anaplastic
Adenocarcinoma	Alveolar cell

Clinical Features

A. **Due to local disease:** Cough, hemoptysis, dyspnea, chest pain, wheeze

B. **Metastatic:**
   1. Intrathoracic
      a. *Nerves:*
         Phrenic: Hiccough, diaphragm paralysis
         Recurrent laryngeal: Hoarseness
         Cervical sympathetic: Horner's
         Vagus: Gastric symptoms
         Brachial plexus: Pain in arm, wasting of small hand ms
         Intercostal: Pain along nerve

b. *Tubes:* Esophagus: Dysphagia
c. *Vessels:* SVC—Venous engorgement of head and neck
Azygos: Dilatation of veins on thorax
Thoracic duct: Chylous effusion
Arteries: Axillary—Loss of peripheral pulse
d. *Bones:* Erosion of ribs with pain and tenderness
e. *Pericardium:* Pericarditis.

2. Extrathoracic
a. *Lymphatic:* Mediastinal and cervical nodes.
b. *Hematogenous:* Intracranial, liver, bone, skin, subcutaneous tissue and muscle.
c. *Bronchogenic:* In same or other lung.

C. **Non-metastatic manifestations:**

Anemia (and thrombocytopenia)

Blood vessels: Thrombophlebitis migrans. Thrombotic endocarditis

Bone: Hypertrophic osteoarthropathy

CNS: Neuromyopathies
1. Encephalopathy, cerebellar degeneration.
2. Neuropathy, proximal myopathy, polymyositis, myasthenia, dermatomyositis

Dermal (skin):
Pruritus
Rashes: Acanthosis nigricans, bullous pemphigoid, herpes zoster

Endocrine

ACTH: Cushing's
ADH: Hypokalemia
Thyroid: Thyrotoxicosis
Parathormone: Hypercalcemia
Estrogen: Gynecomastia

Fall in weight

Growth: Carcinoid tumor.

ACUTE LUNG INJURY AND ACUTE RESPIRATORY DISTRESS SYNDROME

Causes

1. **Respiratory**
   - **A**spiration injury
     Gastric juice
     Chemicals
     Drowning
   - **B**acterial infection: Pneumococcal (also viral)
   - **C**ontusion (pulmonary)
   - **D**isseminated TB
     Drugs: Paraquat, heparin
   - **F**at embolism
   - **G**as (oxygen) toxicity
   - **H**eroin
   - **I**nhalation: Chlorine, nitrous oxide.
2. **Nonrespiratory**
   - **A**cute pancreatitis
   - **B**urns (severe)

- Cardiopulmonary bypass
- DIC
- Exfoliative dermatitis
- Eclampsia
- Failure peripheral (shock)
- Goodpasture's syn.
- General anesthesia
- High altitude
- Infection: cerebral malaria, sepsis syndrome
- Injury (extrathoracic).

Clinical Features

Cough and dyspnea
Cyanosis
Crackles over lung fields.

Diagnosis

X-ray: Diffuse pul. infiltrates (Snow storm).
Blood gas: PaO_2 <4.5 kPa (despite FIO_2 >0.4–0.6).

Management of Cause if Continuing Plus

Assisted respiration
Balance (fluid). Best dry
Cardiac: Monitoring and support, oxygen
Drugs: Antibiotics
Extracorporeal membrane oxygenation.

SEVERE ACUTE RESPIRATORY DISTRESS SYNDROME

Clinical Features

Fever

Symptoms of lower resp. tract infection: Cough, dyspnea, myalgia.

Diagnosis

X-ray chest: Early local infiltrates progressing to more patchy interstitial infiltrates.

Treatment

Antibiotics

Antiviral: Ribavirin + methylprednisolone.

MEDIASTINAL MASSES

Mediastinum	Normal contents	Mediastinal mass
Anterior	Thyroid Thymus Fat Lymph gland	Intrathoracic goiter Thymoma Lipoma Lymphadenopathy TB Sarcoid Hodgkin's Metastatic
Middle	Ascending aorta Pericardium	Aneurysm Cyst

Posterior	Descending aorta Esophagus Intercostal nerves	Aneurysm Cyst Neurofibromas Neurilemmomas Neurogenic sarcomas
	Sympathetic ganglia	Ganglioneuromas Ganglioneuro-blastomas Neuroblastomas
	Lymph nodes	Hilar and Mediastinal lymphadenopathy. Paravertebral abscess.

Masses in Anterior Mediastinum: 4Ts

Thymic masses
Teratomas
Thyroid masses
'Terrible' lymphomas.

FUNGAL LUNG INFECTIONS

1. **Aspergillosis**
   Allergic aspergillosis: Asthma
   Impaction mucoid: Collapse lung
   Mycetoma (Aspergilloma)
   Invasive aspergillosis (in immunocompromised): Local cavitary or disseminated pneumonia.

2. **Actinomycosis:** Clinical features of pneumonia, lung abscess or empyema
3. **Blastomycosis:** Resembling TB but bone involvement more common
4. **Cave fever (Histoplasmosis)**
   Benign pneumonitis like TB
5. **Coccidioidomycosis (Valley fever):** Rapid onset of fever and pneumonic process resemble tuberculosis and histoplasmosis but no miliary form.

Types of Lung Reactions

Asthma
Bronchitis (and tracheitis)
Cancer
Destructive lung changes (resulting in emphysema and chronic airways obstruction)
Edema: Acute pulmonary edema
Fibrosis.

DIFFUSE PARENCHYMAL LUNG DISEASE

Causes

Common

Asbestosis
Blood vessel dis.: Vasculitis
C(S)arcoidosis
Drugs: NFT, bleomycin
Extrinsic allergic alveolitis

Fibrosing alveolitis (cryptogenic)
Growths: Hematological malignancy
Hypertension (chronic pulmonary)
Infection: Viral pneumonia, miliary TB, *Pneumocystis jiroveci.*

Uncommon

Hereditary disorders: Tuberous sclerosis, neurofibromatosis
Histiocytosis X
Hemorrhage syndrome (pulmonary alveolar).

SARCOIDOSIS

1. **Thoracic:** Stages
   Stage I: Hilar adenopathy usually bilateral and symmetrical
   Stage II: Bilateral hilar lymphadenopathy with diffuse bilateral pulmonary infiltrates
   Stage III: Diffuse pul. fibrosis, traction bronchiectasis and cysts.
2. **Extrathoracic:**
   Arthralgia
   Bone involvement (esp. cysts)
   CNS: Cranial nerve palsies
   Cerebral deposits

Meningoencephalitis
Myelitis.

Dermal: Erythema nodosum plaques, lupus pernio
Eyes: Uveitis
Fever: Uveoparotid fever
Glands: Enlarged esp. cervical
Heart: Arrhythmias
Block
CHF
Hypercalcemia (and nephrocalcinosis)
Infiltration of liver and spleen.

PULMONARY EDEMA

Alveolar (Pulmonary)

Infection: Influenza, strepto, varicella

Injury: Chemical: Chlorine, bromine, phosgene, sulfur
Physical: Blast injuries, hot gas
Mechanical: Overhydration, inhalation of gastric contents.

Brain Damage

Morphine, barbiturates, organo P poisoning, head injury, intracranial hemorrhage.

Cardiac: LV failure, MS.

PULMONARY EOSINOPHILIA

Causes

Atopic allergy
  Asthma
  Allergic bronchopulmonary aspergillosis
  Simple pulmonary eosinophilia
Bowel infection (Helminthic): *Ascaris, Schistosoma* spp.
Churg-Strauss syndrome
Drugs: Nitrofurantoin, sulfa, penicillin, minocycline, chlorpropamide, imipramine
E(I)diopathic
  Acute eosinophilic pneumonia
  Idiopathic hypereosinophilic syndrome
Filarial: Tropical eosinophilia.

SLEEP APNEA

Sleep-disordered Breathing

Apnea: Complete cessation of airflow for at least 10 seconds.
Hypopnea: 60% reduction in airflow for at least 10 seconds terminating in arousal.
Obstructive event: Continued resp. effort despite reduced airflow.
Central event: Absent resp. effort with absent airflow.
Hypoventilation: Abnormal rise in $PaCO_2$ during sleep without specific resp. events.

Cheyne-Stokes resp.: Usually seen in heart failure or neurological disease.

Apnea-hypopnea index: >5 usually considered abnormal (except in elderly).

Predisposing Factors for OSA

Obesity
Reduced muscle tone
Gender: Higher incidence in males
Abnormality (genetic craniofacial): Narrowing of upper airway, high arched palate, adenopathy
Nasal obstruction.

RESPIRATORY FAILURE

Types

Type I: Hypoxemic (Normal or low $PaCO_2$)
Type II: Ventilatory (High $PaCO_2$).

Causes

1. **Upper airway obstruction:** Foreign body, obstructive sleep apneas.
2. **Lung disorders:**
   Asthma (severe)
   Bronchitis (chronic)
   Consolidation (Pneumonia)
   Distress syndrome (ARDS)
   Emphysema
   Fibrosing alveolitis.

3. **Respiratory pump failure**
   a. *CNS:*
      Acute cerebrovascular accident
      Brainstem disorders
      Cervical cordotomy
      Drugs: Overdose of sedative drugs.
         Organophosphorus poisoning.
      Encephalitis (Polioencephalitis)
      Fits (Status epilepticus)
      GB syndrome
   b. *Muscles:*
      Myasthenia gravis
      Muscular dystrophies
      Myopathies (congenital)
   c. *Thoracic cage:*
      Crushed chest, kyphoscoliosis, thoracic or upper abdominal surgery.

Clinical Features

Hypoxia: PaO_2 <60 mm Hg (8 kPa)
Confusion
Cyanosis
Compensatory mechanism–Hyperventilation, hypertension.

Hypercapnia: $PaCO_2$ >50 mm Hg (6.6 kPa)
Arrhythmias
Bounding pulse

Cutaneous flush
Confusion and coma
Drowsiness
Diaphoresis
Extensor plantar
Engorged retinal veins
Flap.

Management

Clear airway
Control cause, e.g. antibiotics for septicemia
Concentration of inspired O_2 to be raised
Controlled ventilatory assistance
    Noninvasive, intubation, tracheostomy.

PLEURAL DISEASE

Unexplained Pleuritic Pain: Differential Diagnosis

Pleurodynia (Bornholm's disease)
Pneumonia
Pneumothorax
Pulmonary infarction
Pericarditis
Pancreatitis
Pathologic rib fracture
Phrenic (subphrenic) abscess.

PLEURAL EFFUSION

Causes

Infection: Pulmonary TB, pyogenic organisms, viruses, fungi
Infiltration: Metastasis, mesothelioma
Infarction: Pulmonary
Immune (auto) diseases: RA, SLE, Still's disease
Iatrogenic: Drugs like hydralazine, procainamide, nitrofurantoin, methysergide. Post-coronary bypass
Intra-abdominal: Amebic liver abscess, subphrenic abscess, pancreatitis.

Transudate	Exudate	Hemorrhagic
Acute glomerulo-nephritis (and nephrosis)	**I**nfection: TB, viruses	**I**njury
Beginning of atelectasis (early phase)	**I**nfiltration: (malignant)	**I**nfarction
Cirrhosis of liver	**I**nfarction	**I**nfiltration (TB. Ca)
Dialysis (peritoneal)	**I**mmunological (RA, SLE, Wegener's)	**I**atrogenic
Embolism pulmonary (acute phase)	**I**ntra-abdominal disease (Pancreatitis, subphrenic or hepatic abscess)	
	Idiopathic	
	Irradiation	

Pus	**Chyle**
Infection (local or systemic)	Injury (thoracic duct)
Injury (penetrating)	Infection (TB)
I(E)sophageal rupture	Infestation (filaria)

Signs (Dullness with Silence)

Diminished chest movement, VR
Dull note
Deviation of mediastinum
Decreased breath sounds.

Absence of Mediastinal Shift in Pleural Effusion

Apical fibrosis
Bilateral effusion
Collapsed lung, e.g. malignancy
Diminutive (small) effusion
Encysted effusion.

Differential Diagnosis

Thickened pleura (difficult clinically) and
Amebic liver abscess (rt. side)
Bronchogenic carcinoma
Consolidation. Collapse
Diaphragmatic (subdiaphragmatic) abscess
Empyema

Fibrosis
Growth (pleural mesothelioma)
Hydrothorax.

Indications for Aspiration

Acute pulmonary edema
Bilateral effusion
Clavicle reached by fluid
Dyspnea
Empyema
Failure to respond to medical treatment
Growth suspected
Hemorrhagic fluid
High protein content of fluid.

PNEUMOTHORAX

Causes

1. **Spontaneous:**
   Common:
   Tuberculosis
   Benign spontaneous pneumothorax (rupture of subpleural bleb).

   Uncommon:
   Asthma
   Bronchiectasis

Consolidation (*Staph. pneumoniae*)
Developmental (congenital) cyst
Emphysema (chronic bronchitis)
Fibrosis (interstitial)
Growths (Bronchial and pleural)
Honeycomb lung
Industrial lung disease (especially aluminosis and bauxite lung)

2. **Iatrogenic:** Lung biopsy, positive pressure ventilation, thoracocentesis
3. **Traumatic:** Stab wounds, crush injuries.

Types

Closed
Open
Tension (valvular).

Signs

Hyperresonance with silence
On side of pneumothorax:
Apex beat shift
Bulging of chest
Cardiac dullness obliterated (if left side)
Diminished breath sounds
Expansion of chest diminished.

Management of Pneumothorax

Observation	**Minor symptoms**
Simple aspiration	Significant dyspnea Traumatic (minor)
Large-bore tube drainage (often with suction)	Spontaneous air leak Traumatic (major) Ventilated
Indwelling catheter drainage	Failed simple aspiration
Thoracoscopy/ thoracotomy	Persistent leak Recurrent pneumothorax

Hydropneumothorax

Etiology: Tuberculous till proved otherwise

Signs: Splash (succussion)
Shifting dullness.

CHAPTER

4 Nervous System

VERTIGO

Classification

1. **Peripheral**
   Int. ear: (Otological) labyrinthitis/neuronitis—
      Iatrogenic: Salicylates, strepto, etc.
      Infection, e.g. viral
      Injury (head)
      Ischemia
      Meniere's
      Benign paroxysmal positional vertigo (BPPV)
   Middle ear: Eustachian block, glomus tympanicum, tumor
   External ear: Wax
2. **Central** (Neurological)
   Congenital:
      Ataxia: Friedreich's
      Atrophy: Spinocerebellar
      Arnold-Chiari malformation

Acquired:

Multiple sclerosis

Migraine

3. **General medical causes:**

Vasovagal episodes

Orthostatic hypotension

Low cardiac output, e.g. arrhythmia

Hyperventilation

Duration of symptoms	**Suggested diagnosis**
Several seconds to few minutes	Benign paroxysmal peripheral vertigo, perilymphatic fistula
Several mins to one hour	Posterior TIA, perilymphatic fistula
Hours	Meniere's disease, migraine, perilymphatic fistula from trauma or surgery, acoustic neuroma
Days	Early acute vestibular neuronitis, stroke, migraine, multiple sclerosis
Weeks	Psychogenic (constant vertigo lasting weeks without improvement)

Provoking factor	Suggested diagnosis
Change in head position	Acute labyrinthitis, benign positional paroxysmal vertigo, CFA tumor, MS, perilymphatic fistula
Spontaneous episodes	Acute vestibular neuronitis, stroke or TIA, Meniere's disease, migraine, multiple sclerosis
Recent upper respiratory tract illness	Acute vestibular neuronitis
Stress	Psychiatric causes, migraine
Immunosuppression (drugs, old age, stress)	Herpes zoster oticus
Changes in air pressure head trauma, excessive straining, loud noises	Perilymphatic fistula

HEADACHE

Causes

PMO

A. **Psychogenic**

B. **Muscle contraction** (tension) headache

C. **Organic**

1. *Extracranial (Referred)*
   Arteries: Temporal arteritis
   Bones: Cervical spondylosis
   C(s)inuses: Sinusitis
   Dental: Abscess
   Ear: Middle ear disease
   Eyes: Glaucoma
   Face: Trigeminal neuralgia
2. *Intracranial*
   a. Migraine
   b. Non-migrainous
      Hemorrhage (subarachnoid)
      Hypertension
      Hangover (Alcoholic)
      Hypercapnia
      Hypoglycemia
      Post-seizure
      Post-traumatic
      Pyrexia
      Inflammation: Meningitis
      Infiltration: Tumor
      Iatrogenic: Post-LP
      Increased intracranial pressure.

MIGRAINE

Precipitating Factors

Alcohol
Bright lights (and noise)

Contraceptive pill
Drugs and some foods (Chocolate, cheese)
Emotion
Fatigue
Gestation (Pregnancy)
Hormonal changes (Pre-menstrual).

Types: 3 Cs

Common: Migraine without aura
Classical: With aura—Visual paresthesiae
Complicated variants: Hemiplegic
Vertebrobasilar
Ophthalmoplegic.

Diagnosis: POUND

Pulsating headache
One day duration
Unilateral
Nausea
Disabling in character.

Treatment of Acute Attack

Analgesics: Paracetamol 600 mg, Ibuprofen 400 mg,
Ergotamine 1 mg po q1/2h till max. 3 mg/d.
Prochlorperazine 12.5 mg IM

Triptans:
Sumatriptan: 50–100 mg po
Rizatriptan 5–10 mg po, 6 mg sc, 20 mg nasal spray.

Prophylaxis

1. Elimination of trigger zones
2. Relaxation exercises
3. Drugs:
   a. Serotonin (5-HT) inhibitors
      Flunarizine 10 mg/d
      Pizotifen 0. 5 mg tds or 1.5 mg nocte
      Methysergide 1–2 mg tds
   b. Topiramate 2.5–5 mg bd
   c. Amitriptyline 25 mg tds
   d. Progesterone for premenstrual migraine.

Cluster Headache (Migrainous Neuralgia)

Severe pain usually in one orbit. Redness and watering of ipsilateral eye during attack. Lasts 1/2–2 hours. No aura, vomiting seldom.

Tension Headache

Mild generalized pain without the incapacity, nausea or photophobia associated with migraine.

Treatment

Relaxation and stress management by psychology therapy.

Idiopathic Intracranial Hypertension

Almost daily headache of fluctuating intensity at times with nausea, visual loss, bengins peripherally, diplopia and pulsatile intracranial tinnitus may occur.

Treatment

Lumbar puncture, diuretics NSAIDs. Obese patients must lose weight.

INVOLUNTARY MOVEMENTS

Generalized	Localized
Athetosis	Asterixis (liver flap)
Ballism	Blepharospasm
Chorea	Craft spasm
Dystonias	Dyskinesia (some drug-induced)
Epilepsy	Essential (hands initially)
Flexor (and extensor) spasms	Fasciculations. (Dying cry of a motor neuron)
Tremors:	Facial spasms
Rest (Parkinson's)	
Postural (Essential)	Torticollis (spasmodic)
Action or intention (Cerebellar)	Titubation
	Myoclonus (focal)
Tics	
Myoclonus (general)	

Causes of Chorea

Genetic	Nongenetic
Huntington's disease	Sydenham's
Benign hereditary	Metabolic
Wilson's disease	Chorea gravidarum
Spinocerebellar ataxia type 2	Drug-induced:
Neuroacanthocytosis	Vascular chorea
Dentatorubropallido-luysian atrophy	Infective cause
McLeod syndrome.	Senile chorea

SPEECH

Disorders: 4 Ds

Dysphasia **D**ysphonia
Dysarthria **D**ementia

Aphasia

Types and site:	Features:
Expressive or motor (Broca's) Ant. to central fissure	Non-fluent hesitant speech Telegraphic Good comprehension Poor handwriting
Receptive or sensory (Wernicke's) Parietal and temporal lobes	Speech fluent but nonsensical Neologisms Paraphasias

Global	Non-fluent speech
Large area of dominant hemisphere	Impaired comprehension
Conductive	Speech nonsensical but fluent
Arcuate	Comprehension normal.

Dysarthria

1. **Spastic (Cortical, corticobulbar):** Speech slurred
2. **Ataxic (Cerebellar):** Scanning speech, at times explosive
3. **Flaccid:** X and XII nerve nuclei or nerves—Guttural, nasal speech
4. **Rigid (Extrapyramidal):** Parkinsonism
5. **Myasthenic:** Muscle fatigue, e.g. on asking patient to count.

CRANIAL NERVES

OLFACTORY NERVE (1ST)

Hyposmia

Usually local cause (Also vitamin A deficiency, diabetes)

Anosmia

Injury (Head)
Infections: Common cold

Iatrogenic: Penicillamine
Infiltration: Olfactory groove meningiomas
Increased intracranial pressure
Also aneurysm of circle of Willis.

OPTIC NERVE (2ND)

Site of lesion	Field defect
Optic n.	Central scotoma
Ant. to optic chiasm	Monocular
At optic chiasm	Bitemporal
Behind optic chiasm	Homonymous
Behind lateral geniculate bodies	Congruous homonymous

Pupils

Pupillary Reaction Pathway

Light	Accommodation
Afferent: Optic n.	Arise in frontal lobe

Efferent: Parasympathetic component of 3rd N. on both sides.

Dilated (Mydriasis)

III n. lesion: Ptosis, impaired eye movements
Tonic pupil (Adie's syndrome)
Drugs: Mydriatic drugs. Amphetamine.

Constricted (Miosis)

Normal in young and aged.

Horner's Syndrome

Pre-ganglionic—Pupil dilates after 1% cocaine in eye
Post-ganglionic—No dilatation after cocaine. A–R pupil
Poisoning—Opiates, organophosphorus
Pontine lesion.

Argyll Robertson

Causes
Alcoholism
Brainstem lesions
Cerebral tumor
Disseminated sclerosis. **D**iabetes
Encephalitis
Fracture (Injury behind eyes)
GPI
Herpes zoster ophthalmicus.

Characteristics of AR pupil: 4 As IMM
AR Accommodation retained (light lost)
Anisocoria (unequal)
Atrophy of iris
Absent ciliospinal reflex
Irregular
Miotic
Mydriatic response poor.

Unequal Pupils

Aneurysm of aorta
Bleeding intracranial

Cranial nerves (3rd) palsy
Dementia paralytica
Encephalitis (sometimes).

Fundus

Difference between Papilledema and Papillitis

Examiner sees	Patient sees	Inference
Nothing (cannot find fundus)	Everything	Papilledema
Nothing	Nothing	Papillitis
Everything (normal disc)	Nothing	Retrobulbar neuritis

Common Causes

Papilledema	*Papillitis*
High intracranial pressure	MS, idiopathic
Hypertension (malignant)	
Hypercapnia.	

Optic Atrophy

1. **Primary:** Not preceded by swelling.
   Alcohol (Tobacco-alcohol amblyopia, methyl alcohol)
   Blood vessel: Ischemia of optic nerve, arteritis, anemia
   Congenital (Hereditary): Oxycephaly, Leber's

Degenerative: MS, Tay-Sachs, Niemann-Pick
Endocrine (and metabolic): Addison's, uremia
Fracture of orbit (Optic nerve trauma)
Growth: Orbital, optic nerve glioma, metastasis
H(I)infection: Viral, parasitic, meningitis, post-inoculation.

2. **Secondary:** Pale edges, normal arteries
Monocular sudden visual loss
Arteritis (cranial)
Bleeding (Vitreous hemorrhages)
Cerebrovascular accident
Clotting of central retinal vein
Detachment of retina
Embolism of retinal artery
Faked blindness (Hysterical)
Glaucoma (acute)
Hemicrania (Migraine)
Inflammation (Retrobulbar neuritis)
Injury.

Eye Movements

III, IV, VI Cranial nerves
Control following muscles:
VI: Lateral rectus only
IV: Superior oblique (SO_4)
III; All others.

OCULOMOTOR NERVE (3RD)

- **Aneurysm nerve:** Aneurysm at junction of internal carotid and anterior communicating artery can cause 3rd nerve palsy
- **Herniation nerve:** Herniated temporal lobe.

Paralysis: 3 Ds, 2 Ps

Dilated pupil
Diplopia
Divergent squint
Ptosis
Paralysis of ocular movement.

AR Pupils: 4 Ss

Syphilis (Neuro)
Sarcoidosis
Syringobulbia
Sugar high (DM).

Ophthalmoplegia

External Ophthalmoplegia

Paralysis of extraocular muscle.

Internal Ophthalmoplegia

Paralysis of sphincter pupillae and ciliary muscle.

Causative Lesions of External Ophthalmoplegia

Infranuclear

Myasthenia, mass lesions within orbit, cavernous sinus or near brainstem.

Internuclear

Lesion of medical longitudinal fasciculus
Unilateral: Small pontine infarct
Bilateral: Demyelination.

Nuclear

Vascular or demyelination affecting brainstem nuclei of III, IV or VI Ns.

Supranuclear

Frontal infarcts.

Ptosis

1. Congenital
2. Acquired
   Myasthenia gravis
   Neurosyphilis: Tabes
   Ocular myopathy
   Paralysis of cervical sympathetic (Horner's) or of 3rd nerve.

Pseudoptosis

Tabes
Tumors of eyelids

Diplopia

Brainstem: Infarction, MS
Orbit: Tumor, hemorrhage
Myoneural junction: Myasthenia
Nerve: Neoplasm, infarct, sarcoid
Muscle: Thyrotoxicosis.

Patterns of Doubling

- Horizontal doubling on gaze to right—Weakness of right lateral rectus from right VIN palsy (single nerve, single m., single action turns the eye out).
- Horizontal, vertical and tilted, doubling when reading—IVN lesion. (Single n., single m., complex action brings eye fully down, in and intorted).
- Doubling in most directions, least on looking out—IIIN palsy.
- Variable doubling not of a 'cranial nerves pattern'—Muscular disease, e.g. thyroid orbital disease (diplopia on waking, and myasthenia (later in the day).

Double Vision Rules

1. Diplopia is maximal in direction of gaze of affected muscle
2. False image is the outer image
3. False image arises in affected eye.

Isolated 3rd Nerve Palsy

Accidents: Vascular (upper midbrain)
Base of skull neoplasm
Carotid artery aneurysm
Diabetes
Demyelinating disease
Eye (ophthalmoplegic) migraine.

Horner's Syndrome

Causes

Brainstem: Tumor, vascular, syringobulbia
Cervical cord: Tumor, syringomyelia
Middle fossa: Tumor
Internal carotid artery: Trauma, occlusion
Cervical sympathetic: Pancoast syndrome.

Clinical Features

(Everything gets small and contracts)

Practise	Ptosis
Medicine	Miosis
Ethically	Enophthalmos
Always	Anhidrosis.

TROCHLEAR NERVE (4TH)

Trauma Nerve

Vertex head injury common cause of paralysis.
Movement of eye down and out (copying) impaired.

ABDUCENT NERVE (6TH)

Tumor nerve

Increased intracranial pressure common cause of paralysis
Affected eye turns towards nose.

Nystagmus

Main Types

Pendular: Equal velocity, amplitude in all directions
Jerk: Fast phase, slow phase

1. **Spontaneous**
   a. *Physiological:* Optokinetic
   b. *Peripheral:* Vestibular system in ear, 8th N. nucleus or N.
   c. *Central:* Central vestibular connection or cerebellum
   d. *Retinal:* Inability to fixate
2. **Positional:** Elicited by Hallpike maneuver:
   Nystagmus on postural testing (moving patient quickly from upright to supine position)

	Benign paroxysmal vertigo	**Central vertigo**
Adaption	Disappears in 50 secs.	Persists
Fatigue	Disappears on repetition	Persists
Vertigo	Present	Absent
Direction	To undermost ear of nystagmus	Variable
Incidence	Common	Uncommon

Cranial Nerves V and VI

The Face

TRIGEMINAL NERVE (5TH)

Sensory to

Absent corneal reflex: Early sign of sensory trigeminal lesion
Cornea
Sinus (and nasal mucosa)
Face
Tests: **T**eeth
Tympanic membrane
Tongue.

Motor to

Muscles of mastication
Jaw moves to paralyzed side.

Trigeminal Neuralgia

Sharp stabbing pain
Severe intensity
Symptoms associated: Face in involuntary spasm on affected side with excessive flushing, lacrimation.

Precipitating Factors

Abrupt (Spontaneous)
Blow on face

Chewing
Drinking hot and cold fluid
Exposure to cold wind
Face wash.

Differential Diagnosis of Facial Pain

1. Symptomatic TN:
   Compression from acoustic neuroma, meningioma, Tolosa Hunt syn, MS
2. Referred pain from paranasal sinuses, teeth, temporomandibular joint
3. Vascular pain: Migraine, temporal arteritis
4. Other neuralgias: Post-herpetic, glossopharyngeal
5. Atypical facial pain in depression and anxiety
6. Clonic facial spasm.

FACIAL NERVE (7TH)

Peripheral Function

Face, ear
Taste, tear
Face: Ms. of facial expression
Ear: Stapedius
Taste: Ant. 2/3 if tongue
Tear: Parasympathetic to lacrimal glands

Paralysis

Supranuclear

Present: Movements of upper (supra) part of face
Emotional movements

Nuclear and Infranuclear

Whole face involved.

Site	Cause	Features
Pons	Vascular Demyelinating Tumor Syringobulbia Encephalitis	VI nerve palsy Contralateral muscle weakness
Cerebello-pontine angle or int. aud. meatus	Acoustic neuroma Meningioma Glomus jugulare tumor	V, VIII (XI, X, XI) nerve palsies Loss of taste, salivation, and lacrimation Hyperacusis
Facial canal	Fracture base skull Ramsay Hunt syn. Bell's palsy Carcinoma	Loss of taste and salivation, lacrimation normal
Peripheral nerve (facial ms.)	Parotid gland lesion or operation Trauma	No loss of taste salivation or lacrimation Weakness may be localized

Bilateral Facial Paralysis

Causes

Acute inflammatory polyneuropathy (GBS)
Basal meningitis
C(S)arcoidosis
Diphtheria
Encephalitis
Facioscapulohumeral dystrophy
Gravis (myasthenia)
Hansen's disease
Infection (Double otitis media).

AUDITORY NERVE (8TH)

Cochlear Function

Deafness	Rinne test in deaf ear	Weber test
Conductive	BC > AC	Deaf ear
Sensorineural	AC > BC	Good ear

Cranial Nerves IX, X, XII

GLOSSOPHARYNGEAL (9TH)

The Mouth

Sensory: Posterior 1/3 tongue, pharynx, middle ear
Motor: Stylopharyngeus (cannot be tested)
Autonomic: To parotid.

VAGUS NERVE (10TH)

Weakness of palate
Nasal reg. 'Ah' test: Palate pulled → sound side.
Vocal cord palsy: Bovine cough. Hoarseness.

HYPOGLOSSAL NERVE (12TH)

Weakness-wasting of half tongue (On protrusion moves towards paralyzed side)

Remember:	**SOS**
5th N.	**S**ame side (Jaw)
10th N.	**O**pposite side (palate)
12th N.	**S**ame side (tongue).

ACCESSORY NERVE (11TH)

Weakness-wasting of: Sternomastoid
Trapezius

Note: Ipsilateral cerebral hemisphere supplies contralateral trapezius and ipsilateral sternomastoid. Hence, single UMN lesion can give rise to signs on both sides.

MULTIPLE CRANIAL NERVE PALSIES

Causes

1. **Base of skull**
   Tumors
   Basal meningitis (especially TB)
   Carcinoma

2. **Brainstem:** Infarction, demyelination, MND, syringobulbia, tumors, poliomyelitis
3. **Lower cranial nerves syndromes:** Jugular foramen syn.
4. **Systemic causes:** Diabetes, sarcoidosis.
5. **Idiopathic.**

WASTING OF SMALL MUSCLES OF HAND

A. **Lesion in reflex arc**

1. *Spinal column:* Spondylosis, metastasis, disc
2. *Spinal cord:* Syringomyelia, compression
3. *Ant. horn cell:* Polio, PMA
4. *Nerve root:* Spondylosis, tumor, pachymeningitis
5. *Brachial plexus and peripheral nerve:*
   Amyotrophy (neuralgic)
   Bullet (or stab) wound injury
   Costoclavicular syndrome
   Diphtheria
   Entrapment neuropathy (Carpal tunnel syndrome)
   Leprosy. Lead poisoning
6. *Myoneural junction:* Eaton-Lambert syndrome
7. *Muscle:* **M**uscular dystrophies
   Myotonia atrophica
   Myositis (Poly)
8. *Posterior root ganglion:* Herpes zoster
9. *Posterior root entry zone:* Tabes.

B. **Disuse atrophy**
   Paralysis: Hemiplegia
   Arthritis
   Immobilization.

C. **Systemic disease**
   Diabetes mellitus
   Thyrotoxicosis
   Tuberculosis
   Malignancy.

SENSORY SYSTEM

Dermatomes

C_2	Occiput
C_5	Shoulder
C_7	Middle finger (longest finger and longest C spine)
T_3	Axilla
T_4	Nipple
T_{10}-T_{12}	Abdomen (umbilicus T_{10})
L_1	Ilioinguinal
L_3	Knee
S_1	Small toe
S_2	Perianal
$S_3S_4S_5$	Concentric rings around anus.

Sensory Defects

1. **Cortical:**
   Cortical type sensory loss
   Barognosis

Astereognosis
Graphesthesia

2. **Brainstem:** Loss of pain, temperature on face and opposite side of body (lateral medullary syndrome)
3. **Thalamic:** Total hemisensory loss
4. **Spinal cord:**
   a. *Total transection:* Total loss of all sensations below definite level
   b. *Hemisection:* Loss of pain, temp. opp., JVP same side
   c. *Central cord:* Dissociated anesthesia
   d. *Cauda equina:* Saddle analgesia.
5. **Root:** Variable impairment of sensation in distribution of nerve roots. Pain more affected than touch.
6. **Single nerve:** Sensory loss depending on distribution.
7. **Peripheral nerve:** Glove and stocking anesthesia. Tender calf ms.
8. **Functional:** Glove and stocking anesthesia
   Abrupt demarcation between area of sensory loss and normal sensation
9. **Posterior column:** Loss of JVP with intact pain, temperature.

Dissociated Anesthesia: SALTS

Syringomyelia
Anterior spinal artery thrombosis or hemorrhage

Leprosy
Tumor (intramedullary)
Syndromes: Brown-Sequard, Wallenberg's.

TONE

Decreased (Flaccidity)

UMN lesion	Chorea
Cerebellar lesion	Spinal shock

Increased

Spasticity: UMN lesion
Rigidity (Cog wheel/lead pipe): Parkinson's disease
Paratonia: Bilateral frontal lobe damage, e.g. cerebro-vascular disease
Myotonia: Dystrophia myotonica
Congenital myotonia.

REFLEXES

Ankle	S1
	S2
Knee	L3
	L4
Biceps	C5
Supinator	C5
	C6
Triceps	C6
	C7.

Causes of Absent Deep Jerks

1. **Focal lesion within reflex arc:**
   Anterior horn cells: Polio, PMA
   Anterior nerve root: Tumor
   Motor nerve: Diphtheria, trauma
   Myoneural junction: Eaton-Lambert
   Muscle: Myopathy
   Sensory nerve: Peripheral neuritis, e.g. diabetes
   Posterior root ganglion: Herpes zoster
   Posterior root entry zone: Tabes dorsalis
2. **Lesions outside spinal reflex:**
   Shock (cerebral or spinal)
   Spasticity (and contractures)
   Strained (unable to relax) individuals
3. **Extensor plantar:** Pyramidal tract lesion and
   Apnea
   Blood sugar low
   Coma
   Deep sleep
   E(I)nfancy.

Transient Babinski

Apneic conditions
Autointoxicants
Biochemical disturbances
Convulsions (artificially induced)
Drugs
Epilepsy.

Absent Abdominal Reflex

Physiological: Old age, obesity
Previous abdominal surgery
Pregnancy (repeated)
Pyramidal tract lesion (above that level)
Peripheral nerve lesion or
Posterior column lesion.

Absent Ankle Jerk and Extensor Plantar: FACTS

Friedreich's ataxia
Amyotrophic lateral sclerosis
Conus medullaris lesion
Taboparesis
Subacute combined degeneration.

ABNORMAL GAIT

Neurological

Unilateral:

- Hemiplegic
- High steppage (unilateral)
- Hysterical

Bilateral: 7 Ss and A B C D

Spastic	Spastic paraplegia
Steppage	Peripheral neuritis
Shuffling	Parkinsonism
Stamping	Tabes
Scissors	Cerebral diplegia

Stuttering (marche a petit pas)	Pseudobulbar palsy Alzheimer's Normal pressure hydrocephalus
Springing	Lathyrism
Apraxic	Frontal lobe pathology
Ataxic	Cerebellar, sensory
Bizarre	Functional
Choreiform (Jaunty)	Chorea
Duck-like (Waddling)	Muscular dystrophy

Non-neurological

Painful:	Arthritis
Orthopedic:	Shortened limb Hip surgery.

CEREBROVASCULAR DISEASES

Classification: CVS

Cerebral ischemic disease:
Transient ischemic attacks (TIAs)
Progressive stroke (stroke in evolution)
Completed stroke
Venous infarct
Subarachnoid hemorrhage.

Hemiplegia

Sudden onset: EAT	**Time**
Embolism	Seconds (Bolt from the blue)
Apoplexy	Minutes
Thrombosis	Hours
Slow onset: IT	
Infection	Days
Tumor	Weeks

Risk Factors in Stroke

Alcohol
BP rise
Cigarette smoking
Diabetes
Endocarditis: Valvular heart dis., AF
Fat (obesity)
Geriatrics (Old age)
Hyperlipidemia
Infarct (myocardial).

Stroke Syndromes

Artery and Area Supplied	*Resulting Syndrome*
Internal carotid:	
Middle cerebral	Contralateral: UMN facial

Parietal, frontal, superior temporal lobe	Weakness, hemiplegia (leg > arm), hemianopia, aphasia (dominant hemisphere)
Anterior cerebral	Contralateral leg and foot
Anterior and superior medial frontal lobe	Weakness or hemiplegia (leg > arm), grasp reflexes, incontinence
Vertebrobasilar:	
Posterior cerebral	Contralateral hemiplegia
Occipital lobe	Cortical blindness if bilateral
Inferior temporal lobe	Amnesia especially if bilateral ischemia
Part of thalamus	Contralateral sensory loss Thalamic pain
Posterior inf. cerebellar:	
Lateral medulla	Vertigo and vomiting. Dysphagia
Inf. cerebellum	Ipsilateral cerebellar signs Ipsilateral Horner's Contralateral hemisensory loss below neck
Vertebral and basilar artery:	Diplopia, dysarthria, dysphagia Contralateral hemi or tetraparesis Contra or bilateral sensory loss.

Stroke in a Young Patient

Arteriovenous malformation/aneurysm
Blood vessel dis.—Vasculitis, severe hypertension, dural sinus thrombosis
Cardiac disease—AF, mitral stenosis/valve prolapse, infective endocarditis
Disseminated sclerosis
Epilepsy (Post-ictal)
Functional (Hysterical)
Growth (Intracranial tumor)
Hemicrania (Classical migraine)
Infection—Encephalitis. Neurosyphilis.

Focal Transient Neurological Disturbance

Arterial disease (Cerebrovascular)
Blood diseases: Anemia, polycythemia, sickle cell disease
Clot (embolus) from heart
Disseminated sclerosis
Epilepsy
Functional (Hysterical)
Growths (and other structural intracranial disorders, e.g. chronic subdural hematoma, angioma)
Hemicrania (Migraine)
Hypoglycemia
Hyperviscosity syndrome
Hypertension (malignant).

Recurrent Hemiplegia

Attacks of transient ischemia
Blood sugar fall
Congestive attacks of GPI
Disseminated sclerosis
Encephalopathy (Hepatic)
Functional
Grand mal (Post-ictal)
Hemiplegic migraine.

SUBARACHNOID HEMORRHAGE

Causes

Aneurysm: Usually congenital berry (70%)
A-V malformation
Anticoagulants (and bleeding diathesis)
Idiopathic (No known cause).

Clinical Features

1. **F**ocal signs: Paralysis—Hemi or monoplegia
   Cranial nerve (3rd or 6th)
   Fundus: Subhyaloid hemorrhage
   Fluid (spinal): Blood stained, later xanthochromic
   Fever
2. **Signs and symptoms of increased intracranial pressure:** Headache, nausea, vomiting, stupor, coma

3. **Signs and symptoms of meningeal irritation:**
   Stiffness of neck and spine,
   Kernig's, Brudzinski's.

Complications

1. **Cerebral ischemia and cerebral vasospasm**
   Fifth day after hemorrhage
   Fall in level of consciousness
   Focal neurological signs: Dysphasia, hemiplegia (appears or worsens)
   Fresh hemorrhage absent (Repeat LP)
   Focal areas of low density on CT scan
2. **Hydrocephalus.**

Treatment

Medical: Rest in bed (4 weeks)
Reduction of BP, cerebral ischemia (Nimodipine),
Intracranial pressure.

Surgical: Clipping or wrapping of aneurysm. Ligation of internal or common carotid.

EPILEPSY

Types

1. **Generalized seizures:**
   a. *Tonic-clonic (grand mal) seizures*
      Consciousness lost (with fall)

Contractions (muscular)

Tonic phase (10 seconds) followed by

Clonic phase (1–2 minutes)

Consciousness regained

Confusional state (Post-ictal)

b. *Absence (petit mal) seizures*

Triad: Akinetic seizures

Blank spells

Clonic jerks

c. *Myoclonic seizures*

d. *Tonic, atonic seizures*

2. **Partial seizures:**
   a. *Simple partial:* without impairment of consciousness (Jacksonian, temporal lobe seizures)
   b. *Complex partial*: with impairment of consciousness
   c. *Secondarily generalized*: Partial seizure evolving to tonic/clonic convulsion.

Status Epilepticus

Repeated seizures without recovery in between

- Generalized convulsive tonic-clonic
- Complex partial status epilepticus with prolonged confusion and disorientation with automatic activity
- Partial focal, usually motor (epilepsia partialis continua)
- Non-convulsive or absence.

Conditions that can Mimic Epileptic Seizures

Diagnosis	Important Clinical Features
Hyperventilation	Anxiety and overbreathing
Hemicrania (Migraine)	Visual symptoms prominent
Panic attack	Abrupt onset with feeling of fear, autonomic features
Psychogenic seizures	Psychiatric history. Patient usually motionless Fluttering eye movements
Transient unconsciousness (Syncope)	Syncope with rapid return to normal
Transient global amnesia	Isolated amnesic syncope. No alteration of consciousness
Transient ischemic attack	Sudden onset without progression of symptoms.

Antiepileptic Drugs

Drug	Dosage	Indication
First line drugs		
Carbamazepine Oxcarbazepine	7.5 mg/kg/d (200–800 mg/d)	Partial and tonic clonic seizure

Phenytoin	15–20 mg/kg in status, Maintenance 15–20 mg/d	Partial and generalized tonic-clonic seizures
Sodium valproate	400–800 mg increased by 200 mg/wk. Max 200 mg/d	Progressive myoclonic seizures
Ethosuximide	250 mg increased by 250 mg 15/d	Absence seizures
Second line drugs		
Clobazam	5–20 mg/d	Partial and generalized seizures
Lamotrigine	50 mg od, increase by 50 mg/wk. Max 400 mg/d	Partial and generalized seizures
Vigabatrin	500 mg od increase by 500 mg/q 1–2 weeks Maintenance 1–1.5 g bd	Infantile spasms

Gabapentin	300–400 mg/d Increase weekly by 400 mg, max. 400 mg tds	Can be used as adjunct
Topiramate	25 mg/d, increase by 25 mg weekly to 100 mg bd	Partial and generalized seizures
Zonisamide	100–200 mg/d	All types of epilepsy
Levetiracetam	500 mg bd (max 1,500 mg bd)	As first line or adjunct to partial and generalized seizures

COMA

Causes: 4 Ss

1. **Structural brain damage:**
   Infarction
   Infection: Meningitis, encephalitis, abscess
   Injury: Traumatic hematoma
   Infiltration: Tumor
   Idiopathic: Spontaneous hematoma

2. **Systemic and metabolic disorders:**

Causes	*Clinical Features*
Hypoxia	Slow onset usually
Hypoglycemia	Pupils and eye movements normal
Hepatic (or kidney) failure	Limbs hypotonic
Diabetic ketoacidosis	No focal neurological signs

3. **Sedatives and poisons:**
   Alcohol
   Hypnotics/sedatives
   Organophosphorus and other poisons
4. **Sunstroke.**

Clinical Features

Can result from

1. **Diffuse encephalopathy:** Generalized disturbance of brain function.
2. **Supratentorial lesions**
   - Mass lesions:
     Paresis (hemi)
     Papilledema
     Progressive changes

- Associated with distortion of brainstem (coning):

	Uncal herniation	*Central herniation*
Early	Ipsilateral dilated pupil. Signs and symptoms of supratentorial massive lesion	Erratic respiration Small reactive pupils Increased tone Bilateral Babinski
Later	Ipsilateral hemiplegia Ptosis and III nerve palsy Cheyne-Stokes respiration	Cheyne-Stokes respiration Decorticate rigidity
Still later	Tetraparesis Bilateral dilated fixed pupils Erratic respiration Death	Fixed dilated pupils Decerebrate posturing
Progression	Rapid	Slow

Diagnostic Signs

1. **Limbs:**
   Decorticate: 2 Es—2 limbs (lower) extended
   Decerebrate: 4 Es—All 4 limbs extended

2. **Eye movements:**
   Cerebral lesion: Conjugate deviation of eyes away from hemiplegic side
   Brainstem: Towards hemiplegic side
   Doll's head maneuver:
   a. Eyes move in opposite direction to head movement: Normal
   b. Eyes move to one side only: Lateral gaze palsy: Brainstem lesion
   c. Limitation of movements other than abduction: III nerve palsy
   d. Eyes fail to move in any direction: Bilateral brainstem lesion.
3. **Pupils:**
   Pin point: **P**ontine hemorrhage
   Poisons: Morphine, organophosphorus
   Pyrexia (hyper): Sunstroke
   Fixed dilatation: Brainstem damage
   Small pupils reacting briskly to light: Metabolic cause. (Drug intoxication does not affect light reaction)
   Unilateral dilated: Herniated temporal lobe stretching 3rd nerve.
4. **Respiration**
   Acidotic: Uremia, diabetic coma
   Apneustic: Pontine lesion (Mid or caudal)
   Biot's (ataxic): Medullary dysfunction

Cheyne-Stokes: Bilateral hemispheric dysfunction or metabolic coma
Depressed: Drugs.

Pontine Hemorrhage: 3 Ps

Pin point pupils
Paralysis
Pyrexia.

Causes of Coma as Per Onset Rapidity

Seconds to Minutes

Cerebral hemorrhage
Cerebral infarct (massive)
Subarachnoid hemorrhage
Convulsions (epileptic).

Few Hours

Cerebral infarct or hemorrhage
Acute poisoning (Alcohol, drugs)
Hypoglycemia in diabetics (overdose of insulin or oral drugs).

Hours to Days

Encephalitis, meningitis
Brain tumor
Metabolic or toxic encephalopathies.

Resuscitation: Neurological ABCDEFGHI

Airway : Patient put in recovery position
Breathing : O_2. Artificial resp.
Circulation : Check pulse, BP
Diabetes : Check blood sugar. Dextrose IV if hypoglycemia suspected
Drugs : Naloxone, i.e. if opiate overdose
Epilepsy : Control seizures
Fever : Check for fever, stiff neck
Glasgow : Eye opening, best motor response, coma scale best verbal response
Herniation : As evidence of coning
Investigate further.

Brain Death

Pre-requisites

- Condition result of irremediable brain damage of known etiology
- Deep coma not due to depressant drugs, hypothermia or reversible metabolic or endocrine disturbances
- Stoppage of respiration hence patient maintained on ventilator.

Criteria

Absence of all brainstem reflexes

1. *Pupils*: fixed in diameter and no response to change in intensity of light

2. *Absent*:
   Corneal reflex
   Caloric (oculovestibular) reflexes
   Cough (gag) reflex
   Cranial n. distribution motor responses
   Continued stoppage of respiration on disconnecting mechanical ventilation.

PARKINSONISM

Causes

Idiopathic (paralysis agitans, Parkinson's disease).
Iatrogenic: Phenothiazines, butyrophenone, Rauwolfia alkaloids
Infection: Encephalitis lethargica, syphilitic mesencephalitis
Intoxicants: Methyl-phenyl-tetrahydropyridine, manganese
Injury: Repeated head trauma (Punch drunk syndrome)
Infiltration: Tumor affecting brainstem (very rare)
Inherited (In early onset disease).

Clinical Features of Parkinson's Disease

Tremors (classically at rest)

Rigidity	Flexed simian posture
Lead pipe,	Facial hypomimia
cog wheel	Festinant gait

Presenting Symptoms

Neurological	Psychiatric	Cognition	Non-neurological
Chorea	Depression	Speech difficulty	Muscular and testicular atrophy
Dystonia	Mania	Executive dysfunction	Wt. loss
Rigidity	Psychosis	Short-term memory loss	Osteoporosis
Abnormal gait	Anxiety	Poor attention	Impaired GTT
Eye movement	Suicide tendency	Poor calculation	Heart failure

Drugs for Parkinson's Disease

Drug	Dose	Use
Levodopa/Dopa decarboxylase inhibitor (Carbidopa)	100/25 mg tds	Most effective drug

Dopamine agonists		
Bromocriptine	5–15 mg tds	Less effective than levodopa, but less likely to cause dyskinesias
Pergolide	0.25–1.5 mg tds	
Lisuride	0.2–0.6 mg tds	
Ropinirole	1–8 mg tds	
Pramipexole	0.5–1.5 mg tds	
Anticholinergics		
Kemadrin	*2.5 mg tds*	May help tremor
Amantadine	100 mg bd to 500 mg/day	May suppress dyskinesias
Selegiline	5–10 mg/day	Delays need for levodopa
Catechol-o-methyltransferase inhibitors		
Tolcapone	100–200 mg tds	Reduces predictable motor fluctuations
Entacapone	200 mg with each dose of levodopa	

Surgical Treatment

Thalamotomy	Deep-brain stimulation
Pallidotomy	Transplantation (fetal tissue)

Other Akinetic-Rigid Syndromes

Sydenham's Chorea

Motor impersistence
Inability to sustain eye closure
Wormian tongue
Milkmaids grip
Pronator sign
Tics
Occurs 4–6 months after acute rheumatic fever.

Huntington's Disease

Multisystem atrophy (MSA)
Progressive supranuclear palsy
Diffuse cerebral anoxia
Dystonia musculorum deformans
Spasmodic torticollis.

Wilson's Disease

Clinical features	High tissue copper in
Cirrhosis	Liver
Choreoathetosis	Basal ganglia
Cerebral symptoms (dementia, emotional lability)	Cerebrum
C(K)ayser-Fleischer ring	Cornea
Collecting tubules involvement	Kidneys

Treatment

- Penicillamine 500 mg tds
- Trientine 600 mg tds if side effects with penicillamine
- Zinc acetate 50 mg tds to prevent accumulation of copper (not to be given with penicillamine or trientine)

INTRACRANIAL TUMORS

Bone	: Osteoma
Meninges	: Meningioma
Pituitary gland	: Pituitary adenoma
Pineal gland	: Pinealoma
Cranial nerve	: Neuroma
Blood vessels	: Angioma
Brain tissue	: Glioma
Metastatic	: Bronchus, kidneys, breast.

Clinical Features

1. **Of raised intracranial pressure:**

Psychogenic	Papilledema
Headache	Headache
Never	Nausea
Becomes	Bradycardia
Progressive	Psychological symptoms

2. **Epilepsy:** Focal or generalized

3. **Focal signs of space-occupying lesion**

Frontal lobe:	Mental symptoms Urinary incontinence
Parietal lobe:	Cortical sensory loss
Temporal lobe:	Temporal lobe epilepsy Homonymous hemianopia
Pinealoma:	Parinaud's syndrome (inability to look upward)
Central hemisphere:	Abrupt loss of consciousness but no convulsions
Region of sella:	Bitemporal hemianopia
Infratentorial:	Intracranial pressure rise Cerebellar signs
Cerebello-pontine angle:	Acoustic neuroma
Cochlear:	Deafness
Vestibular:	Vertigo Neurological— Cerebellar ataxia Cranial nerves: V, VII CSF: High protein

4. **Mental changes:** Depression, dementia, apathy.

Increased Intracranial Pressure (ICP)

Causes

Intracranial	Extracranial
Trauma (subdural)	Hypoventilation (hypoxia)
Intracranial hernia	Hepatic failure

Ischemic stroke	**H**yperpyrexia
Hydrocephalus	**H**igh altitude cerebral edema
Hypertension benign intracranial	**I**atrogenic (Drugs, toxins)
Pseudotumor cerebri	**R**eye's syndrome
Post-neurosurgery	**S**eizures
Sinus vein (mega) occlusion.	

Clinical Features of Increased ICP

Cushing's triad (BED)
Bradycardia
Elevated BP
Decreased respiration.

HYDROCEPHALUS

Causes: 4 Is

1. Inherited (Malformation): **5 As**
   - Arnold Chiari deformity
   - Aqueduct stenosis
   - Absence of exit foramina of 4th ventricle (Dandy Walker syndrome)
   - Aneurysm of vein of Galen
   - Arachnoidal cyst
2. Infection: Meningitis (pyogenic, parasitic, TB, fungal)
3. Injury (Ventricular hemorrhage)
4. Infiltration (Neoplasm)
5. Idiopathic (in elderly).

Clinical Features

Neonate/Infant

Appetite poor
Brilliant transillumination
Cracked pot tympany
Dilated scalp veins
Enlarged head
Failure of upward gaze 'Setting sun' sign
Fontanelle tense, fusion of sutures delayed.

Elderly

Normal pressure hydrocephalus (Gait disturbance, dementia, urinary incontinence).

Management of Hydrocephalus

Endoscopy: Communicating hydrocephalus caused by obstruction distal to 3rd ventricle
Shunts

NEUROSYPHILIS

1. **Asymptomatic:** Diagnosed by CSF.
2. **Symptomatic:**
   CPI (congenital and perinatal infection)
   Tabes: CALL
      Charcot's joint
      Ataxia
      Lightning pains
      Loss of sensation

3. **Meningeal**
   Clinical features of meningitis
4. **Meningovascular**
   Cerebral
   Hemiparesis
   Dementia
   Spinal
   Pachymeningitis (cervical)
   Transverse myelitis
   Gumma
   Erb's spinal paralysis.

NEUROTUBERCULOSIS

TB meningitis:	Cerebral spinal
Tuberculoma:	Intracranial spinal
Tubercular abscess	
Tuberculous encephalopathy	With meningitis, without meningitis
Spinal TB	Secondary to Skeletal TB (Pott's disease) Arachnoiditis.

Mechanisms of Spinal Cord Compression

Abscess: Fluid, abscess in spinal cord
Paraspinal abscess
Bone sequestration
Compression of artery in intervertebral foramen

Dislocated vertebrae
Endarteritis
Fibrosis causing ischemia
Granulomatous tissue invading spinal cord or producing spinal compression (Pachymeningitis).

SPINAL CORD COMPRESSION

From Within Outward

1. **Cord:** Tumors
   Extramedullary
   Intramedullary: **WAIT**
      Pains (root)
      Pyramidal signs
      Proteins + (in CSF)
      Wasting
      Anesthesia (dissociated)
      Incontinence
      Trophic changes
2. **Extradural lesions:** Abscess, deposits
3. **Vertebral column: POTTS**
      Pott's disease
      Osteitis deformans
      Tumor
      Trauma
      Spondylosis.

Clinical Features at a Given Level: SLIP Disc

Sensory
Lower motor neuron
Incontinence (Autonomic)
Pyramidal tract signs
Disc: Dorsal roots irritation.

Localization of Segmental Level from Pyramidal Involvement

Above C_4	Spasticity of all 4 limbs
C_2–T_2	Spasticity of lower limbs Flaccid weakness of scattered ms. of upper limbs
T_2–L_1	Spasticity of lower limbs
L_2–S_2	Irregular spasticity of lower limbs Flaccid weakness of scattered ms. of lower limbs.

ACUTE TRANSVERSE MYELITIS

Causes

Parainfectious
- Bacterial: Lyme disease, syphilis TB, mycoplasma
- Viral: Herpes zoster, herpes simplex, influenza, cytomegalovirus, HIV, enteroviruses

Post-vaccinal: Rabies

Systemic autoimmune disease
- SLE
- Sjögren's syndrome

Sarcoidosis
Neuromyelitis optica
Neoplastic (para) syndrome
Multiple sclerosis
Vascular
- Spinal AV malformation
- Iatrogenic: IV heroin
- Thrombosis of spinal arteries.

Clinical Features

Dysfunction of bladder and bowel
Dermatome distribution of pain
Diminished sensation (below level of spinal cord involvement)
Demyelination–Lhermitte's sign.

CRANIOVERTEBRAL ANOMALIES

Types

Arnold-Chiari malformation
Atlas occipitalization
Basilar invagination (Platybasia)
Cervical vertebra fusion (Klippel-Feil syndrome)

Dislocation: Atlanto-axial
Ectasia of cerebellum.

Clinical Features: Syndromes–5Cs

Cervical cord compression
Cranial nerve palsies
Cerebellar signs
Cephalus (Hydro)
C(S)yringomyelia.

Klippel-Feil syndrome Triad: SLR

Short neck
Low hair line
Restricted neck movements.

PARAPLEGIA

Causes of Difficulty in Walking

Absent sensation—Diabetes, Tabes
Basal ganglia dis.—Parkinsonism
Cerebellar disorders
Diminished muscle power
E(I)Involuntary movements, e.g. chorea
Frontal lobe disorders (Apraxia)
Gravis: Myasthenia
Hysterical.

Causes of Paraplegia

Upper Motor Neuron Disorders

1. **Intracranial:** TILT
   Thrombosis
      Of unpaired ant. cerebral artery
      Of sup. sagittal sinus
   Internal hydrocephalus
   Little's disease
   Tumor of falx cerebri
2. **Spinal:**
   Acute Onset

Infection:	Acute transverse myelitis
	Viral, syphilis
	Epidural abscess
Injury:	Fracture dislocation
Infarction:	(or hemorrhage) of ant. spinal artery

   Slow Onset: 4 Ds
   Degeneration of spinal cord
      Amyotrophic lateral sclerosis
      B_{12} myelopathy
      Cervical spondylotic myelopathy
         Craniovertebral anomalies
         C(S)yringomyelia
         Disseminated sclerosis
         Error in development of spinal cord
   Deficiency—Pellagra

Disc: Compression
Dal: Lathyrism.

Lower Motor Neuron Disorders

1. **Ant. horn cell:** Progressive muscular atrophy.
2. **Peripheral nerve:** Peripheral neuritis, Guillain Barre syndrome.
3. **Muscle:** Myopathy.
4. **Myoneural junction:** Myasthenia.

Acute Flaccid Paraplegia

Poliomyelitis
Polyneuritis: Acute inflammatory
Poisoning: Organophosphate, botulism
Periodic paralysis
Potassium loss (Hypokalemia) and Myasthenic crisis.

Chronic Progressive Paraplegia: Always STARTS Slowly

Arachnoiditis
Syringomyelia
Tumors
Ankylosing spondylitis
Radiation myelopathy
Tropical spastic paraplegia
Subacute combined degeneration
Spastic paraplegia (Hereditary).

Brown-Sequard Syndrome (Hemisection of the Cord)

	Ipsilateral	*Contralateral*
At level of lesion	LMN signs Loss of all sensations	Nil
Below the level	Loss of joint, position sense, light touch UMN signs with pyramidal weakness	Loss of pain and temperature

MOTOR NEURON DISEASE

LMN Degeneration

Brainstem	*Spinal cord*
(Motor nuclei of medulla)	(Motor nuclei)
Progressive bulbar palsy	Progressive muscular atrophy
Weakness	Weakness
Wasting of: tongue, palate, pharynx, face	Wasting of: Upper extremities, less often lower
Fasciculations of tongue	

UMN Degeneration

Brainstem	*Spinal cord*
(Corticobulbar tract)	(Corticospinal tract)
Pseudobulbar palsy	Amyotrophic lateral sclerosis

Muscle weakness
Spasticity
Dysphagia
Dysarthria
Diminished tongue movements
Jaw jerk +
Emotional outbursts

Muscle weakness
Spasticity: Lower limbs more than upper extensor plantar

Features of MND

No sensory loss
No bladder disturbance
Not >7 years survival
No affection of ocular muscles

Multiple Levels of Spinal Lesion: ADAM'S Nose

Arachnoiditis
Disc (multiple)
Angiomas
Multiple sclerosis
Secondaries
Nose: Neurofibromatosis.

Combination of UMN and LMN Lesions

1. **Cervical cord compression:** Pachymeningitis, tumor, spondylosis
2. **System degeneration of spinal cord: 5 Ms** **M**yelomalacia (and hematomyelia)

Motor neuron disease
Malnutrition
Multiple sclerosis
Myelopathy due to B_{12} deficiency.

Pure Motor Spastic Paraplegia

Amyotrophic lateral sclerosis
Blood vessel disease: Thrombosis or hemorrhage with recovery of sensory function
Compression (anteriorly placed extradural)
Cerebral palsy
Disseminated sclerosis
Erb's spinal paraplegia
Familial spastic paraplegia
"**G**rains" disease (Lathyrism)
(Rarely subacute combined).

SUBACUTE COMBINED DEGENERATION

Clinical Features

Post. columns
Loss of: Joint sensation and vibration
Sensory ataxia
Rombergism
Pyramidal tracts
Progressive spasticity
Plantar extensor
Peripheral sensory neuropathy
Pernicious anemia.

FRIEDREICH'S ATAXIA

Autosomal recessive
Age: Children 8–15 years
Anarthria
Absent knee and ankle jerks
A(E)xtensor plantar responses
Ataxia of limbs and gait
Anomalies:
  Pes cavus
  Kyphoscoliosis
  Hypertrophic cardiomyopathy.

SYRINGOMYELIA

Atrophy of small muscles of hand
Bulbar palsy (Syringobulbia)
Charcot's joint (and other trophic changes)
Dissociated anesthesia
E(A)ssociated anomalies: Kyphoscoliosis, pes cavus, cervical rib, spina bifida.

Paraplegia with Optic Atrophy

Ataxia (hereditary)
Syphilis
Subacute combined degeneration
Sclerosis (multiple)
Syringomyelia
Pellagra
Infection (Koch's).

Multiple Sclerosis

1. **Clinical features of demyelinating lesions**

Site of demyelination	*Symptoms*	*Signs*
Spinal cord	Limb weakness, Lhermitte's, erectile dysfunction, urinary retention, flexor spasms	Spasticity, pyramidal weakness, lost abdominals, extensor plantar
Brainstem	Ataxia, diplopia, dysarthria, dysphagia, focal weakness	Intranuclear ophthalmoplegia, nystagmus, facial sensory loss, 'rubral tremor'.
Cerebellum	Unsteady gait and slurred speech	Gait and limb ataxia, dysarthria, nystagmus
Optic nerve	Unilateral visual loss and painful eye movements	Lost acuity/color vision, optic atrophy (late)
Cerebrum	Poor memory, personality change, epilepsy	Disinhibition, dementia

2. **Relapsing and remitting course.**

Variant of MND

Progressive Muscular Atrophy

Skeleton hand (muscle wasting)
Absent tendon reflexes.

Progressive Bulbar Palsy

Dysarthria
Dysphagia
Dystonia.

Primary Lateral Sclerosis

Spasticity (slowly progressive)
Weakness of limb (more in legs).

Treatment

1. Modifying course of disease. Interferon beta 1a and 1b, Glatiramer acetate
2. Acute relapse—Methylprednisolone
3. Symptomatic
   a. Spasticity—Baclofen
   b. Incontinence—Oxybutynin.

QUADRIPLEGIA

Spastic

From above downwards

1. **Cortical lesions:**
   Congenital microcephaly
   Cerebrate (Decerebrate) states
   Cerebral palsy

2. **Brainstem lesions:**
   Insufficiency (vascular)
   Infiltration
   Infection: Bulbar polio
3. **Cervical (high) cord lesions:**
   a. *Local:* **Anomaly (Craniovertebral)**
   Blood vessel occlusion
   Compression
   Dislocation (fracture)
   b. *Systemic:* **Sclerosis:**
   Amyotrophic lateral
   Multiple
   Syringomyelia
   Syphilitic amyotrophy.

Flaccid

1. **Within reflex arc:**
   Ant. horn cell: Poliomyelitis (usually asymmetrical)
   Motor nerve: Acute inflammatory polyneuropathy, porphyria, diphtheria.
   Myoneural junction: Acute myasthenia
   Botulism
   Carcinomatous myopathy
   Muscle: Polymyositis
   Periodic paralysis (familial)
2. **Outside reflex arc:**
   Neuronal shock: In brainstem lesion.

CEREBELLAR DISEASE

Lobes and connections	Disorder
Anterior lobe	*Of posture and tone:*
Spinocerebellar	Hypotonia
	Pendular knee jerk
	Past pointing
	Positive Barany's
	Gait ataxia
Posterior lobe	*Of skilled movements*
Ponto-cerebellar	Intention tremor
	Dysmetria
	Dyssynergia
	Dysdiadochokinesia
	Rebound phenomena
Flocculonodular lobe	*Of equilibrium 3Ts*
Vestibulocerebellar	Truncal ataxia
	Titubation
	Tandem gait

Incoordination	Cause
Unilateral	Ipsilateral cerebellar syndrome, e.g. MS, vascular, tumor
Bilateral	Bilateral cerebellar syndrome, e.g. drugs, alcohol, demyelination, degeneration

Nil (Truncal and gait ataxia)	Middle cerebellar syndrome Causes same as bilateral syndrome.

Clinical Features

1. **Of localizing value : Postgraduate Medicine**
   a. **Postural disorders: 3Ps**
      Poor tone
      Past pointing
      Pendular knee jerk.
   b. **Gait disorders: 4Ts**
      Truncal ataxia (seated)
      Tottering (reeling) gait
      Titubation
      Turning towards side of lesion.
   c. **Movement disorders: 5Ds and Rebound phenomenon**
      Dystaxia (intention tremor)
      Dysmetria
      Dyssynergia
      Dysdiadochokinesia
      Decomposition of movement.
2. **Non-localizing: 5 Ss plus nystagmus**
   Skew deviation
   Staccato speech
   Static tremors
   Sluggish jerks
   Stereognosis defective.

ATAXIA

Causes

Multiple sclerosis +
Alcohol
- Wernicke's encephalopathy
- Chronic cerebellar degeneration

Autoimmune
- Miller-Fisher syn.
- Paraneoplastic cerebellar degeneration
- B_{12} deficiency (Subacute combined)

Circulatory
- Cerebellar brainstem hemorrhage/infarct
- A-V malformation

Degenerative (neuro) disease
- Idiopathic late-onset cerebellar ataxia

E(I)nfective
- Encephalitis, often varicella
- Abscess
- Tuberculoma
- Creutzfeldt-Jakob disease
- Tabes dorsalis

Faulty development
- Arnold-Chiari malformation
- Dandy Walker

Growths
- Any primary intracranial neoplasm
- Metastasis

Hereditary
- Spinocerebellar ataxia
- Hereditary motor and sensory neuropathy
- Friedreich's ataxia
- Ataxia telangiectasia
- Ataxia with vit. E deficiency
- Mitochondrial disorders

Iatrogenic
- Lithium
- Phenytoin
- Cytarabine
- Pyridoxine
- Vincristine.

AUTONOMIC NERVOUS SYSTEM

Sympathetic	**Parasympathetic**
ALARM system	HOLIDAY system
Outflow: T_1-L_1	Cr. Ns. III, VIII, IX, X and S_2-S_4
Stimulation causes:	
Tachycardia	Bradycardia
Dilatation of bronchi	Constriction of bronchi
Increased bowel motility	Decreased bowel motility
Inhibition of micturition	Initiation of micturition

Dilatation of pupils	Constriction of pupils
Increase in sweating	Increase in salivation and lacrimation.

Neurogenic Bladder

Frontal bladder	Dementia Strokes Frontal tumors	Urinary urgency, precipitant and uncontrolled voiding of large volumes
Spinal bladder	Trauma MS Tumor	Initially acute retention + overflow incontinence. Later bladder contracts with automatic voiding small volumes of urine
Peripheral neurogenic bladder	Cauda equina lesion: Disc., spina bifida, metastases Peripheral nerve lesion: Diabetes, pelvic surgery, malignancy	Painless distension of flaccid bladder with overflow incontinence and large residual volumes. May be saddle anesthesia Fecal incontinence

PERIPHERAL NERVES

Mononeuropathy

Ulnar Nerve

(Musician's nerve) Lesions of this nerve impair delicate finger movements.

Supplies

1. Flexor carpi ulnaris
2. Flexor digitorum profundus (half).

Median Nerve (Labourer's Nerve)

If damaged, coarse gripping movements and pincer action of thumb and index finger impaired. Supplies the remaining muscles of forearm plus: LOAF

Lateral two lumbricals
Opponens pollicis
Abductor pollicis brevis
Flexor pollicis brevis

Rest of the short ms. of hand are supplied by ulnar n.

Radial Nerve

Lesion causes wrist drop and inability to extend digits.

Sciatic Nerve

Supplies hamstrings
Results in: Loss of knee flexion
Distal foot and leg ms. affected.

Common Peroneal Nerve

Weakness of dorsiflexion and eversion of foot. Foot drop.

Polyneuropathies

Causes

Alcohol

B$_1$, B_6 or B_{12} deficiency

Connective tissue diseases: RA, SLE

Drugs: Isoniazid, methotrexate, nitrofurantoin, vincristine, phenytoin, dapsone, chloroquine, metronidazole

Endocrine (and metabolic): Diabetes, acromegaly, uremia, porphyria

Familial: Peroneal muscular atrophy, hereditary sensory, Friedreich's, Dejerine-Sottas, primary amyloid

Growth (Malignancy)

Heavy metals: As, Pb, Au, Hg

Infections: Leprosy, diphtheria

Inoculations and Injections: Antisera

Inflammatory: GB syndrome

Idiopathic (chronic).

Diagnostic Features

Anesthesia of glove and stocking type

Bilaterally symmetrical

Calf tenderness
Dryness of skin
Depressed deep reflexes (ankle)
Distal muscle wasting
Electromyography (and nerve conduction)
Flaccidity, Foot drop
Gait (high steppage).

Mononeuritis Multiplex

Insufficiency (Vascular): Diabetes, polyarteritis, SLE, RA, Wegener's.
Inflammatory: Leprosy, sarcoidosis
Infiltrations: Malignancy, amyloid
Injury
Immune reactions: Vaccinations, foreign sera and proteins.

Acute Onset Neuropathy

Polyneuropathy acute inflammatory
Porphyria
Poisoning
Postvaccinal
Progressive malignancy

Predominantly Motor

Polyneuritis (G-B syndrome)
Poisoning (lead)

Peroneal muscular atrophy
Porphyria
Pediatric infection (diphtheria).

Predominantly Sensory

Amyloid
B$_1$ deficiency
Cancer
Diabetes
E(He)reditary sensory
Failure (kidney)
Gold (heavy metal)
Hensen's.

Peripheral Neuropathy with Cranial Nerve Palsies

Autoimmune dis. (Polyarteritis)
Barre syn. (Guillain Barre)
C(S)arcoidosis
Diabetes.

Painful Neuropathies

Alcohol, arsenic
B vitamin deficiency
Cryoglobulinemia
Diabetes
E(He)reditary sensory.

Unilateral Foot Drop

Pyramidal lesion (of lower limb)
Peroneal nerve palsy
Prolapsed disc (L5).

Thickened Nerves: CALANDDERS

Charcot Marie Tooth type
Amyloidosis
Leprosy
Acromegaly
Neurofibromatosis
Diabetes
Dejerine-Sottas type
E(I)diopathic
Refsum's syndrome
Sarcoidosis.

DEFICIENCY DISORDERS OF NERVOUS SYSTEM

Thiamine

1. Wernicke's encephalopathy
   Mental symptoms
   Ataxia
   Ophthalmoplegia
2. Neuropathic beriberi

Nicotinic Acid: Psychoneurosis
Spinal spastic syndrome

Pyridoxine:		Convulsions in infancy Polyneuropathy (INH excess)
Pantothenic Acid:		Burning feet syndrome
Vitamin B_{12}:	**C:**	Cerebral: **Mood disorder** **Mental slowness** **Memory defect**
	N:	Neuropathy
	S:	Subacute combined degeneration
Vitamin E:		Ataxia, post. column dysfunction, peripheral neuropathy.

Wasting of Small Muscles of Hand

1. **Cord lesions (C8, T1 level)**
   Motor neuron disease
   Tumor
   Syringomyelia
   Cord compression
   Meningovascular syphilis
2. **Root lesions**
   Cervical spondylosis
   Neurofibroma
3. **Brachial plexus lesions**
   Cervical rib
   Klumpke paralysis
4. **Ulnar or median nerve lesions**
5. **Arthritis of hand or wrist or diffuse atrophy.**

MUSCLE DISEASES

Classification

1. Muscular dystrophy
2. Myasthenia gravis
3. Myositis
   - Suppurative
     Staphylococcus
     Streptococcus
     TB
   - Non-suppurative
     Cysticercosis
     Trichinosis
     Collagen disease
     Myositis ossificans
     Progressive myositis fibrosa
     Myopathy (secondary)
   - Endocrine
     Hyperthyroidism
     Diabetes
     Cushing's
     Corticosteroid therapy
   - Toxic
     Chloroquine
     Alcoholism
4. Miscellaneous
   Hyper- and hypokalemia

Osteomalacia
Glycogen storage disease
Paroxysmal myoglobinuria
Carcinomatous myopathy
Sarcoidosis

5. Muscle atrophy.

MUSCULAR WASTING

Causes

1. **According to reflex arc**
   a. *Primary muscle diseases:*
      Muscular dystrophies
      Inflammatory muscle diseases: Polymyositis
   b. *Ant. horn cell disease:* Motor neuron disease, spinal muscular atrophy
   c. *Root lesions:* Radiculopathy, spondylosis, spinal neoplasms
   d. *Plexopathies:* Brachial plexopathy, diabetic amyotrophy
   e. *Neuropathies:* Axonal, GBS, compression, e.g. carpal tunnel syndrome, infection like leprosy.
   f. *Myoneural junction disorder:* Myasthenia gravis (rare).
2. **Disuse atrophy:** Stroke, cerebral neoplasms, pain following fracture.
3. **Systemic generalized wasting:** HIV, malignancy, thyrotoxicosis, TB.

MYOPATHIES

Genetically Determined Myopathies

Muscular Dystrophies

Muscular dystrophies with predominantly axial and limb girdle weakness.

Duchenne Becker	Muscular hypertrophy particularly of calves Gower's Sign
Emery-Dreifuss Bethlem	Muscular contractures prominent

Limb-Girdle Muscular Dystrophies (LGMDs)

Milder forms: Bilateral scapular winging early feature. Distal involvement and calf hypertrophy variable
Severe forms: present in childhood. Clinically similar to Duchenne muscular dystrophy.

Non-Limb-Girdle Dystrophies with Involvement of Cranial Nerves

- Facioscapulohumeral muscular dystrophy
- Oropharyngeal muscular dystrophy
- Distal myopathies.

Congenital muscular dystrophies present at birth or in first few weeks with proximal weakness and delayed milestones.

Myotonic Disorders

Dystrophic Myotonias

Myotonic dystrophy: Grip and percussion myotonia, plus

- Sternomastoid wasting
- Bilateral ptosis and facial muscle weakness
- Cataracts
- Frontal balding.

Proximal myotonic myopathy: Weakness starts in and is mainly confined to proximal muscles and cramps and myalgias are common.

Non-dystrophic Myotonias and Periodic Paralysis

- Myotonia congenita (chloride channelopathy)
- Episodic weakness (calcium channelopathy)
- Paramyotonia congenita. Periodic weakness (e.g. exercise, exposure to cold)
- Periodic paralyses: Episodic, profound muscles weakness not involving breathing and with normal consciousness and hyperkalemia.

Genetically Determined Metabolic Myopathies

- McArdle's disease: Severe myalgia with cramp soon after exercise. Absent phosphorylase on biochemistry
- Mitochondrial disorders can affect muscle specifically or as part of systemic disease involving CNS

- Malignant hyperthermia characterized by hyperpyrexia, rhabdomyolysis and severe acidosis induced by anesthetic agents.

Acquired Myopathies

Inflammatory Myopathies

Polymyositis: Symmetrical proximal muscles weakness, often associated with myalgia and muscles tenderness

Dermatomyositis: Diagnostic skin lesions—Erythema affecting light-exposed areas

Inclusion body myositis: Usually in those over 50. Indolent in progress, not associated with myalgia but marked muscles weakness.

Myopathies in Systemic Disease

Muscle can be involved directly in infectious diseases, or indirectly through effects of metabolic derangements or immune responses.

Proximal Myopathy

Autoimmune disease (polymyositis/dermatomyositis)
Bone disease (osteomalacia)
Carcinoma
Diabetes (asymmetrical amyotrophy)
Endocrine (Cushing's, thyrotoxicosis)
Familial (Hereditary muscular dystrophy).

Muscular Atrophies (Spinal)

1. **Progressive infantile**
   Acute: Werdnig-Hoffman disease
   Chronic: Childhood Kugelberg Welander disease
2. **Adolescent and adult forms.**

MYASTHENIA GRAVIS

Clinical Features

Ocular: Diplopia, ptosis
Limb weakness: More proximal. Weakness increased by exercise (painless fatigue)
Bulbar muscles: Myasthenic snarl. Difficult speech, swallowing
Respiratory muscles: Breathlessness.

Investigations

Anti-AChR antibody
Anti-striated muscle antibody (in >90%)
A(E)drophonium chloride test.

Myasthenic Crisis

Causes:
Inadequate treatment
Infection
Iatrogenic: Initiation of corticosteroid at high dosage.

Carcinomatous Myasthenia Syndrome

(Eaton-Lambert syndrome)
Exercise improves weakness
EMG: Decreasing action potential with repeated stimulation.

Treatment

1. Thymectomy for thymoma
2. Prostigmin or Mestinon
3. Prednisolone for remission
4. For severe case—azathioprine or mycophenolate mofetil.

Treatment of Myasthenic Crisis

1. Hospitalize
2. Plasmapheresis or
3. Immunoglobulin IV.

Multiple CNS Defects

Causes

Multiple sclerosis
Multiple focal leukoencephalopathy
Multiple infarcts
Multiple metastasis
Meningeal carcinomatosis
Meningovascular syphilis
Also Guillain-Barré syndrome, PAN.

ACUTE ENCEPHALOPATHIES OF CHILDREN

Causes: 6 Is

1. **Infections:**
   Meningitis
   Encephalitis
   Cerebral abscess
2. **Immunization:** e.g. measles
3. **Intoxication:**

Endogenous	*Exogenous*
Metabolic:	Drugs
Inherited, e.g. porphyria	Metals
Acquired, e.g. hepatic or renal failure	Excessive—Salt, water, vitamin A
Endocrine:	Stings
Diabetes, thyroid crisis	

4. **Injury:** Scalds, whiplash injury
5. **Idiopathic thrombocytopenic purpura**
6. **Intracerebral hemorrhage.**

Cerebral Palsies of Childhood: SAD

Spastic
Ataxic
Dyskinetic:
  Choreoathetoid
  Rigid.

CHAPTER

5

Endocrines

SHORT STATURE (DWARFISM)

Achondroplasia and other short-limbed dwarfism
Birth weight low
Caloric (and vitamin D) deficiency
Delayed puberty
Endocrine: Diabetes mellitus, GH deficiency, hypothyroidism, hypoparathyroidism (pseudo)
Familial
Gonadal dysgenesis: Turner's syndrome
Glycogen storage disease
Hurler's disease
Idiopathic hypercalcemia of infancy.

PRECOCIOUS PUBERTY

Causes

Intracranial tumors:
- Hypothalamus
- Mammillary body

Pineal gland
Optic nerves
Brain and cerebellum

Inherited (congenital) malformations:
Stenosis of aqueduct of Sylvius, hydrocephalus, microcephalus, craniostenosis

Injury (post): Perinatal or craniocerebral trauma

Infections (post): Meningitis, encephalitis, syphilis

Idiopathic: Sporadic. Familial
Other causes: Recklinghausen's neurofibromatosis, tuberous sclerosis, idiopathic epilepsy.

DELAYED PUBERTY

	Boys	Girls
	Congenital	*Congenital*
Hypergonadotropic hypogonadism	Klinefelter's Noonan's (Male Turner's) Anorchidia	Turner's Noonan's Ovarian agenesis
	Acquired:	*Acquired:*
	Bilateral castration Orchitis Post-chemo or radiotherapy	Bilateral castration Post-chemo or radiotherapy Autoimmune ovaritis Chronic infection (e.g. TB)

Hypogonadotropic	*Hypothalamus:* Kallman's Prader-Willi Laurence-Moon-Biedl Suprasellar tumors *Pituitary:* Panhypopituitarism Growth hormone def. Post-traumatic	
Simple delay of puberty	Sporadic Familial	
Associated with chronic disease	Cystic fibrosis Chronic kidney failure	Celiac disease Crohn's disease

GYNECOMASTIA

A. **Physiological:** Neonatal
   Senile
   Pubertal

B. **Pharmacological:**
   1. *Estrogen therapy*
   2. *Androgen therapy*
   3. *Binding of estrogen receptors:* Digitalis, griseofulvin, cannabis
   4. *Testicular damage:* Anti-cancer drugs
   5. *Anti-androgens:* Spironolactone, cyproterone acetate, cimetidine
   6. *Mechanism unknown:* Phenothiazines, tricyclics, methyldopa.

C. **Pathological:**
   1. *Increased estrogen production:*
      Adrenal carcinoma
      Bronchial carcinoma
      Cirrhosis of liver
      Dig (Leydig) cell tumors
      Endocrine: Hyperthyroidism
   2. *Decreased androgen production:* Hypogonadism
      a. Hypergonadotrophic: Klinefelter's, castration, orchitis
      b. Hypogonadotropic: Isolated, or part of panhypopituitarism
   3. *Androgen insensitivity:* Testicular feminization
   4. *Other causes:* Leprosy
      Refeeding gynecomastia
      Exfoliative dermatitis.

PITUITARY GLAND

Hormones of Anterior Pituitary

Growth	Growth hormone (GH)
Failure	Follicle stimulating hormone (FSH)
Leads	Luteinising hormone (LH)
To	Thyroid stimulating hormone (TSH)
A	Adrenocorticotropic (ACTH)
Miniature	Melanocyte stimulating (MSH)
Person	Prolactin.

Principal Features of Hypopituitarism

Hypothyroidism (without goiter)
Hypoadrenalism (alabaster skin)
Hypogonadism (crows feet)
Hyposthenuria (diabetes insipidus).

Hyperprolactinemia

Physiological: Pregnancy. Postpartum
Pituitary lesion:
  Tumors
  Stalk lesion: Encephalitis, basal meningitis
Polycystic ovary syndrome
Primary hypothyroidism (severe)
Phenothiazines and other drugs (metoclopramide, methyldopa)
Post-herpes zoster
Periodic self-examination of breasts
Liver/kidney failure.

ACROMEGALY

Clinical Features

Triad due to:

1. **Pituitary tumor:**
   Headache
   Visual field defects
   Cr. N. palsies
2. **GH excess:**
   Arthropathy
   Breast enlargement
   Carpal tunnel syndrome
   Diabetes mellitus
   Enlargement of lips, nose and tongue
   Features coarse
   Field defects
   Goiter
   Hypogonadism
   Hypertension
   Husky voice
   Increased sweating, sebum
   Jaw protrusion (prognathism)
   Kyphosis
3. **Other hormones:**
   Galactorrhea
   Polydypsia
   Variable deficiency of GnRH, TSH, ACTH

DIABETES INSIPIDUS

A. **Cranial diabetes insipidus (CDI):**

1. *Familial:*
2. *Acquired:*

   Idiopathic
   Injury (Head)
   Infection: Meningitis, encephalitis
   Infiltration: Sarcoidosis
   Vascular: Sickle cell, Sheehan's.

B. **Nephrogenic diabetes insipidus (NDI)**

1. *Familial:*
2. *Acquired:*

   Amyloidosis
   Block: Prostate, urethral
   Chronic: Kidney dis. (polycystic, sarcoid, sickle cell)
   Drugs: Lithium, demeclocycline
   E(I)nfection: Pyelonephritis
   Fluid excess (prolonged overhydration)
   Glucosuria
   Hypercalcemia. **H**ypokalemia.

Diagnosis

Urine output >3 liters/24 hours
CDI: Low concentration of plasma vasopressin
NDI: Normal plasma vasopressin.

Polyuria

Causes: 2 Ds 2 Cs 2 Hs

Diabetes: Mellitus
Insipidus

Drugs: Diuretics
Lithium
Demeclocycline

Compulsive water drinking (primary polydypsia)

Chronic kidney failure

Hypercalcemia

Hypokalemia.

Syndrome of Inappropriate Diuresis

Causes

Cancer: Bronchus, pancreas, bladder, prostate. Lymphoma.

CNS lesion: Meningitis, enceph., brain tumor, hemorrhage, injury

Chest: Pneumonia, TB, asthma

Chlorpropamide, chlrothiazide, cyclophos, cyclic (tri.) antidepressants.

Clinical Features

Symptoms of hyponatremia (water intoxication)

Confusion

Convulsions

Coma.

THYROID

Hypothyroidism

Causes

Primary hypo.	**Secondary hypo.**	**Other causes**
Idiopathic **I**mmune (auto) Hashimoto's thyroiditis	Congenital hypopituitary Neoplasm: Pitu. or hypothal.	**I**atrogenic, e.g. amiodarone, lithium, interferon **I**nfiltrative diseases
Irradiation of thyroid	Sheehan's syndrome (Pitu. necrosis)	(e.g. sarcoidosis, amyloidosis, scleroderma, hemochromatosis)
Iodine deficiency **S**ubsequent to Grave's dis. **S**urgical removal of thyroid.		

Clinical Features

Slowing down
Slow speech

Sleepiness
Slow gain in weight
Skin changes (dry or coarse)
Skin pallor
Sluggish bowels
Sensitivity to cold
Slowing of tendon reflexes
Sparse hair.

Diagnosis

Thyroid function—TSH
Total cholesterol
T wave changes (with bradycardia)
Thyroid scan.

Clinical Presentations of Hypothyroidism

Casualty officer—Coma
Cardiologist—Ischemia, CHF, bradycardia
Dermatologist—Dry skin, alopecia
Gastroenterologist—Constipation
Gynecologist—Menorrhagia
Hematologist—Anemia
Neurologist—Polyneuritis, cerebellar features
ENT specialist—Deafness, hoarse voice
Ophthalmologist—Puffy eyes
Psychiatrist—Mental changes
Rheumatologist—Aches and pains, arthritis
Surgeon—Goiter, carpal tunnel syndrome.

Myxedema Coma

Precipitating Causes

Hypoxia
Hypercapnia
Hyponatremia
Heart failure
Infection
Iatrogenic (drugs).

Clinical Features

Hypothermia
Hypoventilation
Hypoglycemia
H$_2$O intoxication
Hallucinations and delusions (myxedema madness).

Hyperthyroidism

Causes: of Thyrotoxicosis

Primary Hyperthyroidism

- Grave's disease
- Toxic multinodular goiter
- Toxic adenoma
- Iodine excess.

Secondary Hyperthyroidism

- Pituitary adenoma secreting TSH
- Trophoblastic tumors secreting HCG
- Gestational thyrotoxicosis.

Thyrotoxicosis without Hyperthyroidism

- Destructive thyroiditis—Postpartum, subacute thyroiditis, amiodarone
- Excessive thyroxine administration.

Clinical Features:

Triad of:	Enlarged gland (Goiter)	
	Eye signs	
	Enhanced metabolism	
Goiter:	Diffuse or nodular	
General:	Weight loss (despite good appetite)	
	Fatigue	
	Sweating, heat intolerance	
Cardiovascular:	Palpitation, tachycardia, atrial fib.	
	Anginal pain	
	Cardiac failure	
Neuromuscular:	Tremors	Myasthenia
	Proximal myopathy	Periodic paralysis
Ocular:	Exophthalmos, stare	
	Lid lag, dry eyes	
	Lid retraction	
	Periorbital edema	
Gastroint.:	Vomiting, diarrhea	
Reproductive:	Oligo- or amenorrhea	
	Infertility, loss of libido	

Skin: Pruritus
Warm moist skin
Hair loss
Onycholysis
Palmar erythema.

Specific for Grave's Disease

Family or personal history of autoimmune disorders (e.g. vitiligo, pernicious anemia, type-1 DM)
Ophthalmopathy
Pretibial myxedema
Thyroid acropachy

Diagnosis: Serum free and total T_4 elevated
[T_4 may be normal and free and total T_3 raised (T_3 toxicosis)]
Serum autoantibodies
Scan of thyroid.

Thyroid Crisis (Storm)

Clinical Features

Tachycardia, delirium, seizure, vomiting, diarrhea.

Treatment

- Carbimazole 600 mg loading, then 100–200 mg/q6h
- Lugol's iodine
- Propranolol
- Dexamethasone
- Cooling
- Treatment of precipitating cause.

Thyroiditis

Acute

Infective: Bacterial, fungal
Irradiation (^{133}I therapy)
Iatrogenic: Amiodarone, lithium, interferon α.

Subacute

Infective: Viral
Silent (including postpartum).

Chronic

Autoimmune: Hashimoto's, atrophic
Reidel's
Infective
Parasitic: Echinococcosis, cysticercosis.

Goiter

Physiological:	**Pathological:**
Puberty	**I**odine deficiency
Pregnancy	**I**diopathic
	Grave's disease
	Goitrogens
	Thyroiditis (Hashimoto's)
	Tumors
	Dyshormonogenesis
	Disorders miscellaneous: TB, Sarcoid, syphilis.

Symptoms of large parenchymatous goiter: 4 Ds

Disfigurement	**D**ysphonia
Dyspnea	**D**ysphagia.

PARATHYROIDS

Hyperparathyroidism

Primary: Adenoma, hyperplasia, carcinoma
Secondary: Increased demand for parathormone due to low calcium
Tertiary: Prolonged secondary hyperparathyroidism from chronic kidney failure or malabsorption

Clinical Features

Stones	Renal calculi. Nephrocalcinosis
Bones	Osteitis fibrosa
	Osteoclastoma
	Osteomalacia
	Cysts
Groans	Peptic ulcer. Pancreatitis
Moans	Mental symptoms.

Hypoparathyroidism

1. Idiopathic
2. Surgical

Clinical Features: 3 Ts 6 Cs

Tetany	**Convulsions**
Tingling	**Cramps**
Trousseau's sign	**Chvostek's sign**
	Cataracts
	Calcification
	Cutaneous changes.

Pseudohyperparathyroidism

Resistance of bone and/or kidney tissue to PTH. Characteristic knuckle sign.

Hypercalcemia

Causes

1. **Parathyroid dependent**
   - Primary hyperparathyroidism
   - Familial hypocalciuric hyperparathyroidism
   - Lithium therapy
2. **Parathyroid independent**
   - Associated with kidney failure
     Secondary hyperpara, milk-alkali syndrome
   - Bone turn over high: Immobilization, hyperthyroidism, thiazide diuretics
   - Cancer (malignancy-related):
     Tumors of lung, kidney
     Local osteolysis: Ca breast, multiple myeloma

- Humoral related:
  D vitamin excess: Vitamin D intoxication. Granulomatous dis: Sarcoidosis, tuberculosis
  Idiopathic hypercalciuria of infancy.

Clinical Features

Anorexia (nausea, vomiting)
Bowels sluggish
Confusion (and drowsiness)
Diuresis (polyuria and polydypsia)
Eyes irritable
Fatigue (Muscle weakness).

Treatment of Severe Hypercalcemia

Additional fluids: Normal saline IV
Buffer: Neutral phosphate buffer IV
Corticosteroids
Diuretics: Frusemide IV.

ADRENALS

Addison's Disease

Common Causes

Autoimmune adrenalitis
Tuberculosis
Bilateral adrenalectomy.

Clinical Features

Anorexia (nausea, vomiting)
Blood pressure low
Cutaneous pigmentation (also muc. mem.)
Decreased
- Energy (fatigue)
- Weight
- Body hair in women.

Diagnosis

Synacthen test

Short Synacthen test: 250 µg IM.
Plasma samples for cortisol at 0, 30, 60 mts
Normal: Cortisol 6 µg/dL
- Rise to 7 µg/dL–21 µg/dL

If test abnormal or equivocal—

Depot Synacthen test: 1 mg depot IM
Blood samples at 0, 1, 4, 8 and 24 hours
In Addison's: Impaired cortisol response throughout.

Emergency Treatment for Adrenal Crisis

Saline	Correction of hypoglycemia
Corticosteroids (IV)	Treatment of precipitant (e.g. sepsis)

Cushing's Syndrome

Causes of excess glucocorticoid

1. **ACTH dependent:** Cushing's disease
   Ectopic ACTH syndrome. Iatrogenic
2. **Non-ACTH-dependent:**
   Adrenal adenoma or Ca. Iatrogenic.

Clinical Features

"Lemon on Matchsticks"

Amenorrhea
Bruising
Cutaneous striae
Calcium depletion (Osteoporosis)
Depression (Psychiatric symptoms)
Diabetes mellitus
Edema
Fat pads: Moon face, buffalo hump, truncal obesity
Growth retardation (children)
Hirsutism
Hypertension
Inability to rise from squatting position
(Proximal myopathy)
Impotence.

Diagnosis

Dexamethasone Suppression Tests

Low dose dexamethasone suppression test:

Dexamethasone 0.5 mg 6 hourly for 48 hours. Serum cortisol measurements at 0 and 48 hours

Suppression of serum cortisol to less than 50 nmol/L: **Normal**

Non-suppression: **Cushing's**

High dose dexamethasone suppression test for cause of Cushing's: Dexamethasone 2 mg 6 hourly for 48 hours. Serum cortisol measured at 0, 24 and 48 hours.

Primary Aldosteronism (Conn's Syndrome)

Hypertension
Hypokalemia
Hypernatremia.

Secondary Hyperaldosteronism

Causes

Renal	Renal (vascular damage)
Hypertension	Hypoproteinemia
Curable	CHF.

Adrenogenital Syndrome (Adrenal Virilism)

Newborn:	Male:	Pseudoprecocious puberty
	Female:	Pseudohermaphroditism
Child:	Precocious puberty	
Adult female:	Virilism	

Pheochromocytoma

Clinical Presentation

Headache
Hypertension (non-paroxysmal in 50%)
Hypotension in 50% (orthostatic)
Heartbeat awareness (palpitation)
Hyperhidrosis.

Signs: 3 Hs

Hypertension
Hypermetabolism
Hyperglycemia.

Diagnosis

Increased excretion of—

Total catecholamines	N: 60 µg/24 hours
Total metanephrines	N: 1 mg/24 hours
Vanilmandelic acid	N: 7 mg/24 hours.

Complications

Constipation
Cardiomegaly
Cerebral hemorrhage
Cholelithiasis
Chronic kidney failure
Carcinoma of thyroid
Cushing's syndrome (ACTH secretion by tumor).

MULTIPLE ENDOCRINE NEOPLASIA

Type	Tumors	Biochemical features
MEN1	*Parathyroids*	Hypercalcemia
	Pancreatic islets	↑ Parathyroid hormone
	• Insulinoma	Hypoglycemia, ↑ Insulin
	• Gastrinoma	↑ Gastrin, basal gastric output
	• Glucagonoma	Glucose intolerance ↑ Glucagon
	• VIPoma	↑ Pancreatic polypeptide
	• Somatostatinoma	↑ Pancreatic polypeptide
	Pituitary (ant.)	
	• Prolactinoma	Hyperprolactinemia
	• GH-secreting	↑ Growth hormone
	• ACTH-secreting	Hypercortisolemia ↑ Adrenocorticotropic hormone
	Associated tumors	
	• Adrenal cortical	Hypercortisolemia or primary hyperaldosteronism
	• Carcinoid	↑ 5-hydroxyindoleacetic acid
MEN2a	*Medullary thyroid Ca*	Hypercalcitoninemia
	Pheochromocytoma	
	Parathyroid	↑ Catecholamines Hypercalcemia ↑ Parathyroid hormone

MEN2b	Medullary thyroid Ca	Hypercalcitoninemia
	Pheochromocytoma	↑ Catecholamines
	Associated abnormalities: **M**ucosal neuromas **M**arfanoid habitus **M**edullated corneal nerve fibers **M**egacolon.	

Other Endocrine Syndromes

- **Polyglandular autoimmune syndromes:**
  Two or more endocrine glands
  Simultaneously hypo- or hyperfunctional
- **POEMS syndrome**
  Polyneuropathy
  Organomegaly
  Endocrinopathy
  M protein
  Skin changes
- **Wolfram syndrome (DIDMOAD)**
  DIDM
  OA
  Deafness.

DIABETES MELLITUS

Classification

1. **Insulin-dependent diabetes mellitus (IDDM)**

2. **Non-insulin dependent diabetes mellitus (NIDDM)**
   Non-obese
   Obese
3. **Malnutrition related diabetes mellitus**
4. **Other types:** Associated with–
   Pancreatic disease, certain genetic syndromes
   Hormonal
   Drug-induced or chemical-induced
   Abnormalities of insulin or its receptors
5. **Gestational diabetes mellitus**
6. **Impaired glucose tolerance:**
   Non-obese
   Obese
   Associated with certain conditions and syndromes.

Hyperglycemia

1. Insulin resistance
2. Increased hepatic glucose output
3. Impaired pancreatic β cell secretion of insulin.

Clinical Features

Polyuria
Polyphagia
Polydypsia.

Complications

All systems affected

1. **CVS:** Hypertension, atherosclerosis

2. **CNS:** Coma

Common:	Uncommon:
Hypoglycemic	Lactic acidosis
Hyperglycemic ketotic	Uremic
Hyperosmolar nonketotic	Nonmetabolic causes

3. **Neuropathy:**

Sensory motor: Acute, chronic

Autonomic:

Arrests (respiratory) during anesthesia, or resp. depressant drugs

Bladder (neurogenic)

Cardiac denervation

Diarrhea

E(I)mpotence

Fall of BP (Postural)

Gustatory sweating.

Mononeuropathy

Entrapment neuropathy (e.g. carpal tunnel syndrome)

External pressure palsies

Spontaneous mononeuropathy, e.g. cranial nerve palsy (usually 3rd and 6th)

Proximal motor neuropathy (diabetic amyotrophy esp. quadriceps)

4. **Renal :** Nephropathy:
   Microalbuminuria

	Persistent albuminuria
	Uremia
5. **Pulmonary**	Tuberculosis more common
6. **Liver**	Hepatomegaly
7. **Ocular**	Cataract, errors of refraction, retinopathy
8. **Skin**	Pyogenic infections
9. **Joints**	Charcot's neuropathic
10. **Sex**	Impotence
	Reduction of fertility and early menopause in females.

Characteristics of Diabetic 3rd Nerve Palsy

Precipitous onset
Painful
Pupillary sparing
Probably reflects microvascular disease of vasa vasorum
Prognosis: Diplopia usually improves within 12 months.

Renal Glycosuria

(Glycosuria in absence of hyperglycemia)
Hurried gastric emptying after gastric surgery
Hyperthyroidism
Hepatic disease
Normal individuals.

Oral Anti-diabetic Drugs

1. **Sulfonylureas**

Gliclazide	5 mg	40 mg
Glimepiride	1 mg	8 mg
Glipizide	2.5 mg	20 mg

2. **Biguanides**

Metformin	1.5–2.5 g/day

3. **Thiazolidinediones**

Pioglitazone	15–45 mg od

4. **Alpha-glucosidase inhibitors**

Acarbose	1 mg tds
Voglibose	0.2 mg tds

5. **Glinides**

Repaglinide	0.5 mg tds
Saxaglinide	60–120 mg tds

6. **DPP-4 inhibitor**

Vildagliptin	50–100 mg/day
Nateglinide	60–120 mg tds.

Insulin

Types

1. Standard recombinant (SR)
   a. Rapidly acting (Actrapid)
   b. Intermediate acting (NPH)
   c. Mixture of a and b (Mixtard)

2. Human insulin analogue
   a. Very rapid acting (lispro aspart)
   b. Intermediate acting mixtures
      Lispro-protamine + Lispro Aspart protamine + Aspart
   c. Long acting (Glargine Detemir ultra 100 g).

Indications

- Type 1 DM
- Gestational diabetes
- Hyperglycemia despite maximum doses of oral agents
- Decompensation due to infection, acute injury or stress
- Severe hyperglycemia with ketosis
- Perioperative before surgery
- Kidney or hepatic disease.

Diabetic Ketoacidotic Coma

Clinical Features

Due to:

1. *Ketosis*	Acetone odor Air hunger Abdominal pain
2. *Fluid and electrolytes low*	BP low Clouding of consciousness Dehydration

Differential Diagnosis

	Ketoacidosis	Hypoglycemia
Pptd. by	Infection	Exercise
	Injury	Evading meal
	Insulin omission	Excess insulin
Abrupt onset	No	Yes
Acetone	Yes (with glycosuria)	No
Breathing	Deep and rapid	Stertorous
Babinski	No	Bilateral
Convulsions	Nil	May occur
Depth of coma	Usually rousable	Deep coma
Dehydration	Marked	Nil
Diaphoresis	Nil	Marked

Management

- **Fluids:** Isotonic saline (liters)

1	Immediately
2	Over 1 hour
3	Over 2 hours
4	Over 4 hours
5	Over 8 hours

- **Insulin:** Continuous IV infusion of rapidly acting insulin 5–10 U/h or im regular insulin 20 U loading dose and 5 U/h.
- **Potassium:** Continue at 10–40 mmol/h until ketoacidosis has cleared.

- **Alkali:** If severe acidosis (pH <7). 50–100 mmol/L of sodium bicarb. in 0.45% saline over 30–60 mts.
- **After 8–24 hours:** Continue IV 0.45% saline with/without 2.5 or 5% glucose as needed. After ketoacidosis has cleared (blood pH >7.35, serum ketones negative), switch to subcutaneous insulin.

Comas in DM

1. Ketoacidotic hyperglycemic
2. Hyperosmolar hyperglycemic state
3. Lactic acidosis
4. Hypoglycemia
5. Kidney failure.

HYPOGLYCEMIA

Causes

1. **Postprandial (Reactive)**

   Endogenous hyperinsulinism: Insulin antibodies, Noninsulinoma, pancreatogenous hypoglycemia Congenital disorder of enzymes of carbohydrate metabolism
   - Galactosemia
   - Hereditary fructose intolerance
   - Others:
     Alimentary hypoglycemia
     Idiopathic postprandial hypoglycemia.

2. **Postabsorptive (Fasting)**
   - Illness (critical)
     Hepatic, kidney or cardiac failure
   - Iatrogenic (drugs)
     Insulin or insulin secretagogues
     Sulfonylureas
     Salicylates
   - Hormonal deficiency
     Cortisol, GH or both
   - Glucagon and epinephrine in DM1
   - Endogenous hyperinsulinism
     Insulinomas
     Autoimmune hypoglycemia
     Antibodies to insulin
   - Others
     Non-beta cell tumors
     Hypoglycemia of infancy and childhood.

Clinical Features

Due to—

1. **Cerebral dysfunction (Neuroglycopenic):**
   Triad of:

Confusion	**A**nxiety
Coma	**B**lurred vision
Convulsions OR	**C**onfusion
	Diplopia. **D**ysarthria
	Epileptic fits

Facial (Perioral) tingling
Generalized weakness
Headache
Ischemic attacks
(Transient paresis)

2. **Excessive adrenaline (Adrenergic): 5 Ps**
   Palpitation
   Perspiration
   Pupils dilated
   Pulse bounding
   Polyphagia.

Hypoglycemia without Hyperinsulinemia

Ingestion of food (Post-prandial)
Ingestion of alcohol
Infection esp. *Pl. falciparum*
Increased exercise
Islet cell (non-islet) cell tumors—Mesothelioma, hepatoma, adrenal Ca.
Iatrogenic: Oral hypoglycemic drugs, postpolyagastrectomy, salicylism (in children), propranolol.

Mn of Addictive Disorder Co-occurring with DM: 5 Ds

Delay the use
Distract yourself
Drink water
Deep breathing
Discuss with someone.

CHAPTER

6 Renal Disorders

PROTEINURIA

1. **Physiological: All Ps**
   Postural (Orthostatic or benign)
   Prolonged exposure to cold
   Protein rich meal
   Pregnancy
   Premenstrual
   Psychological strain
2. **Pathological:**
   Pre-renal : **F**ever
   Fluid (Ascites)
   Failure (CHF)
   Renal : **N**ephritis
   Nephrosis
   Necrotizing lesions of kidneys, TB
   Post-renal : Pyelonephritis
   (Pseudo-proteinuria).

HEMATURIA

Causes: 3 Ts 3 Cs 3 Is

Tumors	Calculus	Infection
Trauma	Cystitis	Iatrogenic
Tubercle	Cysts	Induced by exercise

Acute Retention of Urine

Neurological : Both UMN and LMN lesions
Obstruction : Urethra: Stricture, trauma
Bladder neck: Prostate
Bladder: Stones, tumors
Psychological

Frequency and Nocturia

Anatomical: Prostatic hypertrophy, urethral stricture
Bladder tumor
Cystitis and other UTIs, e.g. urethritis, prostatitis
Disseminated sclerosis.

Urinary Incontinence

1. **Non-neuropathic:** Stress most frequent. Also–
   Antisocial: Brain failure
   Bed-wetting: Reduced awareness
   Chronic retention with overflow
   Dribbling of urine: Postprostatectomy, neuropathic bleeding.

Drugs: Hypnotics, diuretics

E(u)rge: Detrusor instability—Chronic retention with overflow
Hypersensitivity—Infection, stone, TB

2. **Neuropathic:**

Suprapontine	Stroke, tumors, Parkinsonism
Cord	MS, spinal cord injury
Peripheral	Diabetic neuropathy

3. **Extrasphincteric:**
   Fistulas (uretero-or vesico-vaginal)
   Ectopic ureter, epispadias.

KIDNEY FUNCTION TESTS

1. **Glomerular filtration rate (GFR)**
   Serum urea and creatinine concentration.
   Interpretation:
   Creatinine clearance: If <15 mL/minutes—dialysis

Plasma Creatinine	**Plasma Urea**
Raised:	*Raised:*
Large muscle bulk	Reduced GFR (including dehydration)
Acute rhabdomyolysis	GI bleeding
Reduced tubular secretion (K-sparing diuretics, trimethoprim)	Corticosteroid/tetracycline
Catabolic state	
High protein diet	

Reduced:	*Reduced:*
Small muscle mass	Liver disease
Pregnancy	Starvation
Raised antidiuretic hormone	Pregnancy
	Raised antidiuretic hormone

2. **Tests of tubular function:**
   - *Proximal tubular function:* **Type II RTA**
     Urine glucose and aminoaciduria, phosphaturia and low molecular weight proteinuria
     Plasma phosphate and urate
   - *Distal tubular function:* **Type I RTA**
     Urine concentrating ability:
     Sp. gravity
     Osmolality of urine samples over 24 hours
     Urinary acidification (significant acidosis if low plasma bicarbonate and urine pH >5.5).

KIDNEY BIOPSY

Indications

Proteinuria

Proteinuria with renal impairment or asymptomatic if >2 g/24 hours.

Nephrotic syndrome in patients <1 year or >10 years of age

Persistent proteinuria (and hematuria) with renal impairment.

Kidney Failure

- Acute if urinary sediment contains RBC casts or if persisting for more than 4 weeks
- Chronic with normal-sized kidneys to determine prognosis and plan treatment.

Renal Allograft Dysfunction

Systemic disorders, e.g. SLE.

Contraindications

Atrophic kidneys (or single kidney)
Blocked (obstructed) kidney
Coagulation defect
Different size (asymmetrical kidneys)
E(I)nfection (acute urinary)
Failure to control BP
Genetic: (developmental) cystic kidney, hemangioma
Reflux nephropathy.

Complications

A-V fitsula
Blood loss
Damage to (loss of) kidney
E(I)nfection

False biopsy—Inadvertent of liver, spleen, pancreas, intestine.

GLOMERULAR DISEASE

Clinical Manifestations

1. Asymptomatic proteinuria
2. Asymptomatic hematuria
3. Acute nephritic syndrome

   Etiology:

   Infection: Group A strepto, pneumo, viral

   Allergen

   Connective tissue disease, e.g. SLE

   Clinical Features:

   Urinary: Hematuria, proteinuria (mild), impaired GFR

   Edema: Facial and/or ankle

   Hypertension

   Progress: Recovery in 90%.
4. **Nephrotic syndrome**

   Causes: Idiopathic in over 80%. Also–

   Allergy (to insect bites, vaccine)

   Block (Mechanical)

   - Thrombosis of renal vein
   - Renal artery stenosis

   C(S)ystemic diseases: SLE, PAN, Henoch-Schönlein

Drugs (and toxins): Penicillamine, heroin, ACE inhibitors, gold, rifampicin, NSAIDs

Endocrine (and metabolic): Diabetes mellitus, Amyloid

Familial: Airport's, Fabry's, congenital

Growths: Carcinoma, sarcoma, lymphoma (and leukemia)

Hemopoietic: Sickle cell disease

Infections:

Malaria	Syphilis
Hepatitis	Strepto-Staphylo
Herpes zoster	Schistosomiasis

Lupus nephritis

Clinical Features:

Triad of—

Proteinuria (>3.5 g/day)

Hypoalbuminemia

Edema.

Complications:

Hypovolemia

Hyponutritional state

Hyperlipoproteinemia

Hypercoagulability (venous and arterial thrombosis)

Hypocalcemia

Hypercholesterolemia

Higher risk of infection

High serum triglyceride levels producing acute appendicitis or pancreatitis.

Management:

Antibiotics, anticoagulants

Blood (pack cells) or plasma

Corticosteroids

Diet: Protein rich, less salt

Endoxan

Frusemide (or other diuretics)

5. **Rapidly progressive GN:** corresponds to 'crescentic' GN

   Commonest cause—Antineutrophil cytoplasmic antibody-associated vasculitis
6. **End stage chronic kidney failure**
7. **Hypertension.**

URINARY TRACT INFECTION

Factors Predisposing to Infection

Incomplete Bladder Emptying

Abnormal pelviureteric drainage

Obstruction, reflux, polycystic disease, horseshoe kidney

Bladder emptying incomplete:

Neurogenic: Spina bifida, MS, spinal injury

Obstruction: Prostatic hypertrophy, urethral stricture

Bladder diverticula, reflux disease

Calculi
Diabetes (also pregnancy)
E(I)nstrumentation: Bladder catheter, ureteric stents
Fistula: Vesicoenteric.

Pathogenic (Uro) Organism

E. coli, *Proteus* spp., *Klebsiella*.

Persistent Organism

Renal: Scar, stone, papillary necrosis, polycystic kidneys
Ureter: Vesicoureteric reflux. Pregnancy
Bladder: Catheter, prolapse, neurogenic bladder
Urethra: Prostatomegaly, prostatitis.

Factors in Females

Rectal contamination
Urethra short
Stasis (urinary during pregnancy)
Trauma (Coitus and parturition).

Acute Pyelonephritis

Clinical Features

Ache in loins and suprapubic areas
Blood stained urine
Constitutional symptoms: Fever with rigors, malaise
Dysuria (with frequency of micturition).

Treatment

Ample fluids
Alkalinization if severe dysuria
Antibacterial agents, e.g. Levofloxacin 500 mg bd.

Chronic Pyelonephritis

Presentation: 4 Ps

Periodic episodes of urinary tract infection
Pressure (hypertension)
Proteinuria
Progressive kidney failure

Pyuria-*Causes:*

Infection (UTI including TB)
Interstitial nephritis (including analgesic nephropathy)
Infiltration (neoplasm)
Iatrogenic—Catheterization, urinary tract surgery
Intra-abdominal inflammation (appendicitis)
Infants (and children) with fever.

Sterile Pyuria

Infection: TB, chlamydial urethritis
Inadequate treatment of UTI
Immune organism: e.g. *Strep. morbili, Corynebacteria*, etc.

Inflammation of lower tract: Prostatitis, chemical cystitis (cyclophosphamide)

Inflammatory non-infective disease: Calculi, papillary necrosis, interstitial nephritis, polycystic disease.

URINARY CALCULI

Stone type	**Causes**
Calcium oxalate or phosphate	Hypercalciuria Hyperuricosuria Hyperoxaluria High urine pH Low urine vol.
Triple phosphate	Urinary infection with bacteria that possess urease
Uric acid	Hyperuricosuria (also low pH, low volume)
Cystine	Cystinuria.

Hypercalciuria

Causes: Hyperparathyroidism and also

Acidosis: Distal renal tubular

Bone lysis

C(S)arcoidosis

Decubitus (Immobilization)

E(I)diopathic

ACUTE KIDNEY FAILURE

1. **Pre-renal**
   Arterial (renal) obstruction
   Bleeding. Bacterial shock
   Cardiac: infarct, failure
   Diarrhea
   Emesis (vomiting)
   Fitstulae (gut)
2. **Renal**
   Acute glomerulonephritis +
   Acute tubular necrosis: 4 Ps

Postoperative	Pigment release (transfusion)
Poisons	Pregnancy related

   Interstitial nephritis
   Vascular: Large vessel occlusion, accelerated hypertension, vasculitis
   Hematological: Myeloma, hemolytic uremic syndrome
   Others: Hepatorenal syndrome, rhabdomyolysis, acute cortical necrosis.
3. **Post-renal**
   Obstruction: Ureteric or bladder.

Clinical Features

Stages

1. Onset
2. Oliguric

3. Diuretic
4. Recovery

Oliguric stage: Uremia: Retention of—

Sodium and water: Edema. Hypertension. CHF

Urea

Alimentary: Anorexia, nausea, vomiting, diarrhea, GI bleeding
Bleeding
Cardiac: Pericarditis
Drowsiness coma
E(I)nfection
Focal neurological signs: Muscle twitchings
Generalized pruritus

Potassium: Muscular weakness. Arrhythmias

Acid: **R**etching
Restlessness
Respiration hissing

Hematological changes: Anemia
Bleeding

Contributory factors of anemia:
Aluminum toxicity
Blood loss
Curtailed RBC survival
Deficiency of iron/folate, erythropoietin
E(I)nhibition of erythropoiesis
Fibrosis of marrow due to hyperparathyroidism.

CHRONIC KIDNEY FAILURE

Causes

1. Glomerulonephritis (chronic)
2. Interstitial nephritis (chronic): All Is
   Infection (Pyelonephritis)
   Iatrogenic: Analgesic nephropathy
   Intoxication: Metals: Pb Cd Cu
   Infiltration: Neoplasm
   Insufficiency: (Vascular) Renal arterial stenosis
   Inherited disease: Polycystic disease
   Irradiation: of kidneys
3. Other causes
   Pancreatic insufficiency (diabetes)
   Polycystic kidneys
   Papillary necrosis
   Polyarteritis nodosa
   Pressure raised (hypertension).

Clinical Features

All systems affected

GI : **A**norexia
Bleeding (from gums)
Catarrhal stomatitis
Diarrhea
Emesis
Foul odor (uriniferous) of breath
Glandular: Parotitis. Pancreatitis
Hiccup

Skeletal	: **O**steoporosis
	Osteomalacia (or rickets)
	Osteitis fibrosa cystica
CVS	: **A**rrhythmias
	Blood pressure (high)
	CHF, cardiomyopathy
	Dry pericarditis
Eyes	: **R**ed eyes
	Retinopathy (hypertensive)
	Retinal detachment
Pulmonary	: **E**dema (and uremic lung)
	Effusion
	E(I)infection.

Nervous System

Mental disturbances (uremic encephalopathy)

Motor disturbances: Slurred speech, asterixis, twitchings, tremors, myoclonus, seizures, coma

Neuropathy

Skin	: **P**ruritus
	Purpura
	Pigmentation
Psychiatric	: **M**ania
	Anxiety
	Depression
	Delusions

Endocrine : **Gynecomastia**
Hypogonadism (with sterility and impotence)

Hematological : **Anemia**
Bleeding.

Management

Conservative

Acidosis—Sodium bicarbonate
Blood pressure—Diuretics, ACE inhibitors
Calcium supplements—Calcium carbonate and/or aluminum hydroxide
Diet—Restrict proteins, phosphates. Adjust Na, K
Emesis—Domperidone
Fluids—Aim for urine output 1500–2000 mL/24 hours

Renal Dialysis. *Indications:*
Acidosis: pH <7.15
Blood urea >200 mg/100 mL (33 mmol/L) or rising >100 mg daily
Calcemia (hyper) uncontrollable
C(K)alemia (hyper): >7 mEq/L
Drug intoxication: Barbiturates, salicylates, ethanol
Electrolyte disturbance (severe)
Failure: Acute kidney (patient in poor condition) or chronic kidney (acute exacerbation or permanent)
Fluid overload.

Acute dialysis: If hyperkalemia, fluid overload, acidosis and uremia unresponsive to other treatments.

Peritoneal dialysis: Complications—

Mechanical Effects

Abdominal wall hernia
Back pain
Chest problems
Displacement (malposition of) catheter
E(I)ncreased vascular insufficiency
Fluid leaks: Edema of external genitalia, hydrothorax.

Metabolic Complications

Amino acid and protein losses
Appetite loss (from glucose absorption)
Added weight (and hyperlipidemia)
Membrane (peritoneal) damage
Infection.

Hemodialysis

Complications

Arrhythmia
Blood loss (usually minor)
Circuit disconnection: May lead to major blood loss or embolism

Dialysis disequilibrium
E(I)nfections
Fall of BP
General reactions to dialyzer: Anaphylaxis, bronchospasm, fever.

Kidney transplantation: Treatment of choice for ESKF

Contraindications

Age
Associated conditions–that might deteriorate with immunosuppression, e.g. bronchiectasis, severe cardiovascular disease
Antibodies (cytotoxic) to transplant antigen present in high titers.

DRUG-INDUCED RENAL DISEASE

Adverse effects	**Drugs**
Acute tubular necrosis	Aminoglycosides
	Amphotericin B
	Cisplatin
	NSAIDs
	Paracetamol (poisoning)
Crystalluria	Acyclovir
	Methotrexate
	Sulfonamides

Glomerulonephropathy	Membranous: Captopril, gold salts, heavy metals, penicillamine, phenytoin, troxidone Minimal change: NSAIDs Acute nephritis: Penicillins
Interstitial nephritis	Allopurinol Azathioprine Frusemide NSAIDs Penicillins Sulfonamides Thiazides Vancomycin
Nephrogenic diabetes insipidus	Lithium Demethyl chlortetracycline
Renal papillary necrosis	Aspirin NSAIDs
Renal tubular acidosis	Aminoglycosides Amphotericin B Nitrofurantoin.

CHAPTER

7 Hematology

ANEMIAS

Iron Deficiency Anemia

Causes

1. **Inadequate intake**
2. **Inadequate production** of normal red cells
3. **Excessive loss:**

GI tract:	*Genitourinary:*
Peptic ulcer	Menorrhagia
Piles	Recurrent hematuria
Parasites	

4. **Deficiency:** Iron, vitamin B_{12}, folate
5. **Toxic factors:** Chronic infection, kidney failure, hepatic failure, drugs
6. **Endocrine disease** Hypothyroidism, hypopituitarism
7. **Marrow invasion/failure:** Leukemia, secondary Ca, aplastic anemia

8. **Increased demand:**
   Puberty
   Pregnancy and lactation
   Periods (menstruation)
9. **Excessive destruction of RBCs:** Hemolytic anemia.

Clinical Features

1. **Due to anemia:** Lassitude, fatigue, weakness.
2. **Due to tissue effects of iron deficiency:**
   Atrophic gastritis and achlorhydria
   Bald tongue (Glossitis)
   Cardiac: Angina, palpitation, dyspnea. Dynamic circulation. Hemic murmur. CHF. C(K)oilonychia.
   Dysphagia (Plummer-Vinson syndrome)
   Enlargement of spleen (mild)
   Fundal hemorrhages
3. **Due to underlying disease:** Hiatus hernia, piles, etc.

Megaloblastic Anemia

Causes: Deficiency of

Vitamin B_{12}

Inadequate intake: Vegans, malnutrition.

Intrinsic factor deficiency: Pernicious anemia, gastrectomy, congenital intrinsic factor deficiency

Intestinal (small) disease: Bacterial overgrowth (blind loop syndrome)

Crohn's disease, tropical sprue, fish tapeworm. Miscellaneous, e.g. HIV, severe pancreatic disease, drugs like colchicine, neomycin.

Folic Acid

Impaired absorption:

- *Gastric:* IF deficiency in pernicious anemia, post-gastrectomy
- *Intestinal*: Malabsorption, ileal resection, small bowel bacterial overgrowth (e.g. diverticulosis), tropical sprue, Crohn's disease, drugs, e.g. metformin

Increased requirement: Pregnancy

Inadequate intake: Malnutrition, elderly, alcoholism

Increased requirement: Pregnancy, infancy, hemolytic anemias, malignancy

Impaired utilization: Folic acid antagonists

Increased loss: Combined folic acid and B_{12} deficiency–Hemodialysis, tropical sprue, gluten sensitive enteropathy (Non-tropical sprue).

Other Causes of Megaloblastosis

Congenital: Lesch-Nyhan syndrome, homocystinuria, dyserythropoietic anemia.

Acquired (Disorders of DNA synthesis):

- Myelodysplastic disorders
- Metabolic inhibition: (a) Purine (azathioprine, 6-mercaptopurine, aciclovir). (b) Pyrimidine (azarudine). (c) Deoxynucleotide (hydroxyurea, cytosine arabinoside). (d) Others–cyclophosphamide, azidothymidine.

Diagnosis

Blood picture

Bone marrow

Biochemical changes

Raised: LDH, iron, bilirubin

Blood levels (B_{12}, folate).

Sideroblastic Anemia

Sideroblast = Normoblast containing iron granules.

Causes

Inherited: X-linked males.

Acquired

- Idiopathic refractory anemia with sideroblasts
- Secondary:
  Alcohol INH, pyrazinamide, cycloserine

Insufficiency : Malabsorption
Megaloblastic anemia (nutritional)

Infiltration : Myeloproliferative syndrome
Myelomatosis

Anemia of Chronic Disorders

Causes

Inflammation (chronic): RA, SLE

Infections (chronic): TB, chronic bronchitis, UTI, pelvic inflammatory disease, HIV

Infiltration: Lymphomas, malignancy of various organs

Idiopathic

Alcoholic liver disease.

Hemolytic Anemia

A. **Hereditary** (Intrinsic RBC abnormality)

1. Defects in red cell membrane
   Spherocytosis — Stomatocytosis
   Elliptocytosis — Acanthocytosis
2. Defects in globin synthesis
   Thalassemias
   Hemoglobinopathies
   Sickling syndromes
   Unstable Hb disease

3. Enzyme deficiency
   Of glycolytic pathway: Pyruvate kinase deficiency, hexokinase deficiency
   Of G-6-PD
   Of red cell nucleoside metabolism
   Pyrimidine-5-nucleotidase—
   Hemolytic disease of newborn

B. **Acquired** (Extrinsic RBC abnormality)
   1. Immunohemolytic anemias
      Autoimmune: Idiopathic, due to warm or cold antibodies, paroxysmal cold hemoglobinuria.
   2. Fragmentation syndromes: Hemolytic uremic syndrome, DIC, thrombotic thrombocytopenic purpura, prosthetic cardiac valves.

Paroxysmal Nocturnal Hemoglobinuria

Drugs and chemicals
Drugs: Oxidant drugs, dapsone, primaquine
Chemicals: Naphthalene, nitrates and nitrites
Thermal injury and infections: Burns, *Clostridium perfringens, Cl. Welchii* septicemia, cholera
Others: Celiac disease, vitamin E deficiency.

Clinical Features

Splenomegaly
Jaundice
Leg ulcers
Gallstones
Skeletal abnormality

Laboratory Findings

Increased RBC Breakdown

Increased serum bilirubin, urine urobilinogen
Decreased haptoglobin.

Increased RBC Production

Reticulocytosis
Erythroid hyperplasia of bone marrow
Low serum folate.

Red Cell Damage

Shorter red cell survival
Increased osmotic fragility
Morphological abnormality, e.g. fragmentation.

Special Features of Intravascular Hemolysis

Hemoglobinemia
Hemalbuminemia (Meth.)
Hemoglobinuria
Hemosiderin in urine.

Congenital Disorders of Blood Cells

1. Congenital neutrophil disorders
2. Congenital disorders primarily affecting platelets
3. Hereditary RBC disorders
4. Hemoglobinopathies.

HEMOGLOBINOPATHIES

1. **Sickle cell anemia**
   Aplastic crises (and sickling)
   Bone necrosis (aseptic)

Chronic leg ulceration
Damage to kidney, liver (cirrhosis)
Erection painful (Priapism)
Fundal changes: Vitreous hemorrhages, retinal detachment
Gallstone formation
Hypertension: Pulmonary
Infection esp. pneumococcal

2. **Sickle cell trait**
3. **Sickle cell** Hbc (SC) disease.

Types of Sickle Cell Crisis

Hemolytic: Associated sepsis or G6PD deficiency
Aplastic: May signify parvovirus infection or folate deficiency
Thrombotic: Commonest. May affect abdomen, lung, brain
Sequestration: Most serious, especially in infants Rapid onset hepato/splenomegaly

Thalassemias–α and β.

α Thalassemia

- Silent carrier state
- α thalassemia trait: Mild microcytic hypochromic anemia
- HbH disease: Variable anemia with splenomegaly
- Hydrops fetalis.

β Thalassemia

- Thalassemia major (Cooley's anemia):
  Progressive anemia with hepatosplenomegaly
  Small stature and bone deformities
- Thalassemia intermedia: Less severe disorder, usually not transfusion dependent
- Heterozygous β thalassemia: Mild microcytic, hypochromic anemia.

APLASTIC ANEMIA (PANCYTOPENIA)

Acquired

Idiopathic
Iatrogenic
  Drugs: Chloramphenicol, NSAIDs, carbimazole, etc.
  Chemicals: Benzene, arsenic
Infections: Viral hepatitis
Ionizing radiation.

Inherited

Fanconi's anemia
Others: Sideroblastic anemias, myelodysplastic syndromes.

PURE RED CELL APLASIA

Congenital

Diamond-Blackfan syndrome: Cleft/high arched palate, ear abnormalities, flat nasal bridge.

Acquired

- Autoimmune: SLE, NHL
- Thymoma associated
- Viral: Hepatitis, EBVP, arbovirus B_{19}
- Drug-induced: Chloramphenicol, azathioprine, procainamide
- Associated with TB
- Idiopathic.

Clinical Features

Due to deficiency of:

Red cells	Anemia
White cells	Pyrexia
	Ulceration
	Sore throat
	Sweats
Platelets	Bleeding

Bone marrow: Hypocellular. Normal hemopoietic cells replaced by fat cells.

Treatment

Aetiological factor: Determination and treatment

Bone marrow transplantation

Correction of anemia, neutropenia, and thrombocytopenia with blood products

Drugs: Androgens
Anti-thymocyte and antilymphocyte globulin

Human hemopoietic growth factors (G-CSF, GH CSF).

Hemopoietic stem cell transplantation.

LEUKOERYTHROBLASTIC BLOOD FILM

Myelofibrosis
Marrow infiltration
Metastatic Ca (breast, prostate, small-cell lung)
Malignant lymphoma
Melanoma
Marble bone disease (Osteopetrosis)
Metabolic: Gaucher's disease.

Eosinophilia

Causes: Tropical eosinophilia +
Allergic conditions: Asthma, hay fever
Blood disease: Hodgkin's, eosinophilic leukemia
Collagen vascular disease, RA, Churg-Strauss syn.
Drugs: Sulfonamides, nitrofurantoin
E(I) diopathic eosinophil syndrome
Filaria (and helminthic infections).

BLEEDING (HEMORRHAGIC) DISORDERS

Causes

1. Coagulation defect
2. Platelet defect
3. Vascular defect.

Clinical Features

Spontaneous bleeding
Severe bleeding (after trauma or surgery)
Site more than one.

Coagulation Disorders

Congenital	**Acquired**
Hemophilia A	Anticoagulants
Hemophilia B	Blood transfusion (massive)
Von Willebrand's disease	Coagulation disseminated intravascular
	Deficiency of vitamin K and Liver disease.

Hemophilia

Severity of Hemophilia

Factor VIII plasma level	**Clinical defect**
• >50%	Normal
• 20–50%	Abnormal bleeding after severe injury or surgery
• 5–20%	Abnormal bleeding after minor injury or surgery
• 2–5%	Abnormal bleeding after trivial injury Occasional spontaneous bleeding

- <2% — Spontaneous bleeding into joints and muscles
  Severe bleeding after injury or surgery.

Platelet Disorders

Normal platelet count—150–450 x 10^9/L

Thrombocytopenia:

1. Increased platelet destruction:
   a. *Immune mechanisms:*
   Idiopathic
   Iatrogenic: Quinine, quinidine, gold
   Infections: HIV, infectious mono.
   Immunological disease: SLE
   b. *Non-immune mechanisms:*
   Massive transfusion
   Sepsis
   TTP
   DIC and
   Hemolytic uremic syndrome
   Hemophagocytic syndrome
   Hemoglobinuria (paroxysmal nocturnal)
   Hypersplenism
   Hemangioma (giant)
   HELLP syndrome in pregnancy (hemolysis, elevated liver enzymes and low platelets)

2. Decreased platelet production:
   Acquired
   Alcohol toxicity
   Bone marrow aplasia
   Cancer (Bone marrow infiltration)
   Deficiency (Vitamin B_{12} or folate)

   Congenital:
   Absent radii syndrome
   Anemia of Fanconi
   Aldrich-Wiskott syndrome
   Anomaly (May-Hegglin).

Idiopathic Thrombocytopenic Purpura

Treatment

Acute:
Mild: No treatment
Severe: Prednisolone 1 mg/kg/day

Chronic:
- Prednisolone 1–2 mg/kg/d x 2 months
- If not effective or side-effects, splenectomy

For future recurrences:
- Prednisolone
  If no effect:
- Immunoglobulin IV 400 mg/kg x 5 days
  Endoxan 3 mg/kg/d
  or Injection Vincristine IV 1.5 mg/m² body surface once weekly.

Vascular Disorders

Causes

1. **Inherited:**
   Hereditary hem. telangiectasia (HHT)
   Ehlers-Danlos syndrome
2. **Acquired:**
   Septicemia
   Steroids
   Senility
   Scurvy
   SLE (also PAN)
   Skin disease: Eczema, lichen planus
   Systemic disease—
      Allergic (Henoch-Schonlein)
      Amyloid
      Bad nutrition (malnutrition)
      Cushing's
      Drugs and chemicals
      E (I) infection: Bacteria, viruses, rickettsia.

Clinical Features

Hemorrhage	Skin, GI, Venipuncture sites
Thrombosis	Thrombophlebitis
	Gangrene or Cyanosis
Organ failure	Cardiorespiratory
	Kidney
	Jaundice

Diagnostic Features of Bleeding

	Coagulation	**Platelet/Capillary**
Family history	+ve	-ve
Sex	M > F	F > M

Clinical Features

Type of bleed	Visceral	Skin and mm
Onset after trauma	Delayed	Immediate
Bruising	Often large	Usually small
Pressure	Ineffective	Usually effective

Laboratory Findings

Screening tests	APTT (N 25–40) PT (N 12 sec)	BT (N 3–7 sec)

DISSEMINATED INTRAVASCULAR COAGULATION

Causes

Common

Sepsis
Obstetrical complications: Antepartum hem., retained placenta, amniotic fluid embolus. Eclampsia
Malignancy
Hypovolemic shock
Less common:
Hepatic failure
Hypoxia

Heat exhaustion
Injury
Immune response: Incompatible blood trans., anaphylaxis
Iatrogenic: Surgery.

Clinical Features

Adult resp. distress syndrome
Bleeding: Skin, GI tract
Clotting: Cerebral infarct, ARF
Delirium and coma.

Treatment

Heparin: If organ damage, deep vein thrombosis
Coagulation factors: Fresh frozen plasma, platelet concentrates.

Inhibition of excess fibrinolysis:
Aminocaproic acid
Aprotinin.

LEUKEMIAS

Acute Leukemias

Etiological Factors

Irradiation
Iatrogenic: Drugs and chemicals
Infection: Viral
Inherited (Genetic): Down's syndrome.

Clinical Features

1. **From marrow failure:** Leucopenia, anemia, thrombocytopenia.
2. **From accumulation of leukemic cells:**
   Splenomegaly and hepatomegaly
   CNS invasion: Meningeal involvement (more in children)
   Marrow cavity: Bone pain.

Investigations

Count: WBC total, diff.
Coagulation screening
Chest radiograph
Cytochemistry (and immunophenotyping of antigens)
Cytogenetic and molecular studies
CSF

	ALL	AML
Lymphadenopathy	More common	Less
Gum hypertrophy	Yes	No
Hepatospleno.	More	Less
CNS invol.	75% of children	Less common

Management

Phase	**ALL**	**AML**
Induction	Vincristine Prednisolone L-asparaginase or Daunorubicin Dasatinib (if Ph +ve)	Daunorubicin Cytosine arabinoside

CNS prophylaxis	Methotrexate (intrathecal)	
Consolidation	High dose methotrexate 6-thioguanine Dacarbazine	Dasatinib (high dose for 2–3 cycles)
Maintenance	Prednisolone Vincristine 6-mercaptopurine Methotrexate	Myeloablative therapy followed by BMT in those with high-risk chromosomal change

Chronic Leukemias

Cl. Features	CML	CLL
Anemia	Prominent	Slight
Bleeding	May occur at onset	Later stage
Constitutional symptoms	Weight loss, pallor, dyspnea	Not prominent
Deposits		
Bone	Common	Rare
Skin	Uncommon	Common
Enlargement of		
Spleen	90%	In late stage
Liver	About 40%	Late stage
Fever	Prominent	If infection
Glands	Slight in late stage	Presenting features

Investigations		
WBC	>30% x 109/L Neutrophils Myeloblasts	>10 x 209/L Lymphocytes
Bone marrow	Granulocytic hyperplasia. Megakaryocytes+ Ph chromosome	Infiltration by lymphocytes
Course of Disease		
	Chronic phase may progress to accelerated phase	Remission for many years, or relentless increase in tumor load.
Treatment		
	Imatinib mesylate 400 mg/d. In case of resistance: Dozatinib or Nilotinib or Ponatinib	*First line* Chlorambucil Fludarabine CHOP *Second line* Fludarabine Campath IH Methyl prednisolone Others: Splenectomy

Splenic
irradiation
Leukapheresis.

LYMPHOMAS

Hodgkin Lymphoma

Clinical Features

Anemia: Due to bone marrow involvement
Bone pain
Constitutional symptoms: Weight loss, night sweats
Deposits: Extradural (cord), meninges, brain
Excessive itching (pruritus)
Fever: Remittent or Pel-Ebstein
Glands: Often presenting symptom—neck, mediastinum
Hepatosplenomegaly
Infection: Herpes zoster (during therapy)
Jaundice: Usually preterminal.

Management

ABVD

Drug	Dose	
Adriamycin	25 mg/m^2	
Bleomycin	10 units/m^2	IV days 1 and 15
Vinblastine	6 g/m^2	IV days 1 and 15
Dacarbazine	375 mg/m^2	IV days 1 and 15

Give 12 cycles with 2 weeks rest between end of one course and beginning of next

IFRT (Involved field radiotherapy) to all sites of bulky disease post-ABVD.

Non-Hodgkin lymphoma

Etiology

Infections: Bacterial (*H. pylori*) Viral (E-B virus)
Immunodeficiency: Post-transplant, HIV
Immune (auto) disorders
Ionizing radiation
Intoxicants: Carcinogenic chemicals
Inherited: Ataxia telan., xeroderma pigmentosum, Fanconi's syndrome, Bloom's syndrome.

Clinical Features

1. **Lymphadenopathy:** Painless, single node, enlarged regional nodes, or widespread lymphadenopathy
2. **Systemic symptoms:** Night sweats, malaise, weight loss
3. **Extranodal disease:** Skin, lung, bowel, liver, bone marrow, bone, testis
4. **CNS:** Cranial nerve palsies, nerve root and meningeal involvement by deposits.

Management

Indolent (Low grade): 'Wait and watch'

Unless: B symptoms, bone marrow failure, bulky disease, progression—Chlorambucil or Cyclophos or Fludarabine or CVP or CHOP.

R-CHOP in B cell NHL and CHOP alone in T cell NHL (commonly but other regimens can be used depending on type of lymphoma).

R-CHOP

Rituximab	378 mg/m^2	
Cyclophosphamide	750 mg/m^2	per day
Adriamycin	50 mg/m^2	per day
Vincristine	1.4 mg/m^2 (maximum 2 mg)	per day

Given every 21 days x 6 cycles
Response depends on type of lymphoma
R_x Bendamustine in follicular + mantle cell NHL
In high grade lymphoma CNS prophylaxis. Systemic high dose and/or intrathecal methotrexate.

POLYCYTHEMIA (ERYTHROCYTOSIS)

Primary: Polycythemia vera (Spleen+)
Secondary: (No splenic enlargement)

1. **Hypoxic:**
   Altitude. Abnormal Hb (meth). Apnea (sleep)
   Body weight increase
   Cyanotic cong. heart, Cor pulmonale

2. **Erythropoietic:** Tumors: Renal Ca, hepatoma, cerebellar hemangioblastoma, uterine fibroids
3. **Miscellaneous:** Polycystic kidneys, post-kidney transplant.

Polycythemia Vera

Raised hematocrit (>0.51 in men, >0.48 in women)

Clinical Features

1. **Due to hyperviscosity and/or hypervolemia:**
   Cerebral: Headache, dizziness, cerebral thrombosis
   Cardiovascular: Angina, CHF, thrombophlebitis
2. **Due to hemopoietic proliferation:**
   Plethora
   Gout
   Splenomegaly or hepatosplenomegaly
3. **Multifactorial:** Pruritus. Peptic ulcer. Hemorrhages.

Management

Repeated venesection (PCV <0.45)
Low dose aspirin for microvascular occlusion
Hydroxyurea
Radioactive P and intermittent low-dose busulfan (for elderly).

MULTIPLE MYELOMA

Malignant disease of plasma cells in bone marrow.

Clinical Features: CRAB

Hyper**C**alcemia
Renal dysfunction
Anemia
Bone lytic lesions.

Due to–

1. **Plasma cell proliferation:**
   - **Anemia**
   - **Bone pain**
   - **Crush fractures**
   - **Hypercalcemia symptoms**
2. **M-proteins:**
   - Hyperviscosity: Malaise, cardiac failure, confusion, dilatation of retinal veins
   - Beeding tendency
   - Raynaud's phenomena
   - Coagulation abnormalities
3. **Multifactorial:**
   - Renal impairment: Bence Jones proteins
   - Peripheral neuropathy (e.g. Carpal Tunnel Syndrome)
   - Infection particularly chest.

Diagnostic Criteria:

1. Paraproteins in blood and/or urine
2. Marrow infiltration by malignant plasma cells
3. Osteolytic bone lesions (skull, ribs) on X-ray.

Management

1. Combination therapy
   Bortezomib + Lenalidomide + Dexamethasone or
   Bortezomib + Thalidomide + Dexamethasone
   Other drugs used –
   Melphalan + Liposome + Doxorubicin + Cyclophosphamide
2. Bisphosphonates to inhibit bone lysis
3. Stem cell transplantation.

BLOOD TRANSFUSION

Indications

For use of blood and blood products.

RBCs

- Acute blood loss
- Anemia
- Bone marrow failure
- Thalassemia
- Exchange transfusion: Neonates with hemolytic disease of the newborn. Adults with sickle cell disease, severe falciparum malaria.

Fresh Frozen Plasma

- Acquired coagulation defects
- Plasma exchange in thrombotic thrombocytopenic purpura

- Inherited coagulation defects if no specific coagulation factor concentrate.

Platelets

- Therapeutic transfusion in patients who are bleeding: Platelet count <50 × 10^9/L, following massive transfusion with dilutional thrombocytopenia, platelet dysfunction due to drug (aspirin), dengue fever or congenital platelet disorders
- Prophylactic transfusion in thrombocytopenia: Acquired bone marrow failure due to bone marrow disease or chemotherapy/radiotherapy, to cover surgery in thrombocytopenic patients.

Cryoprecipitate

Acquired coagulation defects with clinical evidence of bleeding, chronic kidney failure, inherited platelet function disorders, inherited coagulation defects if no specific coagulation factor concentrate.

Complications of Blood Transfusion

Allergic reaction
Bitis (Thrombophlebitis)
Cardiac overload
Destruction of donor cells (ABO incompatibility)
Embolism: Air (now rare)
Febrile reaction
Graft versus host disease
Hemosiderosis
Infections: Hepatitis, malaria, viral infections, AIDS.

Exchange Transfusion

Indications

- Thrombotic thrombocytopenic purpura
- DIC
- Guillain-Barré syndrome
- Goodpasture syndrome.

BONE MARROW EXAMINATION

Indications

Marrow Aspirate

Anemia: Refractory, leukoerythroblastic, sideroblastic
Blood malignancy: Leukemia, lymphoma, myeloproliferative disease, myeloma
Cytopenias: Neutropenia, thrombocytopenia
Dysplastic (myelo) disorders
E(I)nfection: Malaria, kala-azar, tuberculosis
Fever of unknown origin

Bone Marrow Trephine

Cellular marrow
Dry tap
Fibrosis of marrow
Focal involvement by malignant cells.

Dry tap. Causes
Myelosclerosis
Myelofibrosis

Malignant infiltration of marrow
Marrow heavily infiltrated, e.g. leukemia, lymphoma, myeloma.

SPLENOMEGALY

Causes

HICCUPS

Hematological	: Hemolytic disorders Malignancy (Leukemias, Hodgkin) Polycythemia
Infections	: Bacterial Viral Protozoal Rickettsial Fungal Parasitic
Congestive	: CHF Constrictive pericarditis Cirrhosis (portal hypertension)
Collagen disease	: SLE, Felty's
Unknown etiology	: Tropical splenomegaly
Primary tumors (rarely secondary)	
Storage diseases	: Gaucher's, Niemann-Pick.
Sarcoidosis	

Degree of Enlargement

Massive (>8 cm)	**M**yeloid leukemia (chronic) **M**yelofibrosis **M**alaria (and kala-azar) **M**etabolic disease (e.g. Gaucher's) **H**istiocytosis and TSS
Moderate (4–8 cm)	**A**ll above + **H**emolytic anemia **H**ypertension (portal) **H**odgkin (and other lymphoproliferative diseases)
Mild (4 cm)	**A**cute malaria **B**lood disorders (polycythemia vera, ITP, SLE) **C**(S)arcoidosis **D**isseminated TB **E**ndocarditis (and other infections, e.g. typhoid) **F**elty's syndrome.

Medical Indications for Splenectomy

Hematological diseases:
- ITP
- Malignant lymphoma
- Hereditary spherocytosis
- Chronic granulocytic leukemia

- Acquired hemolytic anemia
- Myelofibrosis

Hydatid cyst

Hypersplenism causing symptoms.

HYPOSPLENISM

Causes

Splenectomy
Sickle cell disease
Systemic lupus erythematosus
Senile atrophy (rare)
Celiac disease (adult)
Crohn's disease
Congenital absence
Cytopenia (Essential thrombocytopenia).

CHAPTER

8

Infectious Diseases and Infections

INCUBATION PERIODS

Short (<10 days)

Acute gastroenteritis
Adenoviral infections (Dengue, chikungunya)
Anthrax
Respiratory tract infections
  Bacterial, viral, influenza
Rickettsial infections (e.g. tick typhus).

Medium (10–21 days)

Bacterial: Enteric fever, brucellosis, leptospirosis, Q fever
Fungal: Coccidioidomycosis, histoplasmosis
Protozoal: Malaria (*Pl. falciparum*), Chagas disease (acute), trypanosoma rhodesiense
Viral: CMV, EBV, HIV, viral hemorrhagic fever, Ebola.

Long (>21 days)

Bacterial: Tuberculosis, brucellosis

Protozoal: Amebic liver abscess, malaria, visceral leishmanias, trypanosoma gambiense
Viral: HIV, viral hepatitis
Fluke: Katayama fever.

MEASLES

Clinical Features

Fever and
Cough
Coryza
Conjunctivitis
Cutaneous rash
C(K)oplik's spots

Complications

Early

Pneumonia
Otitis media
Laryngotracheobronchitis
Encephalitis.
Gingivostomatitis
Hepatitis

Late

Bronchiectasis
Encephalitis—
a. Immunosuppressive measles encephalopathy
b. Subacute sclerosing panencephalitis.

Unusual Forms

1. Modified forms
2. Atypical: 6–14 years after inactivated measles vaccine given previously
3. Hemorrhagic.

RUBELLA

German Measles (3 Day Measles)

Catarrhal Stage

Fever, headache conjunctivitis, mild lymphadenopathy (suboccipital).

Exanthematous Stage

Rash pink macular (lasts about 3 days)
Lymphadenopathy (generalized).

Complications

- Encephalitis
- Intrauterine growth retardation
- Abortion (spontaneous)
- Thrombocytopenia
- Congenital rubella syndrome
  Congenital heart disease (PDA with or without PS)
  Microcephaly
  Cataract.

Late Features

Delayed growth
Deafness
Deficiency (immune)
Hepatosplenomegaly
Myocarditis
Interstitial pneumonia
Mental retardation.

WHOOPING COUGH (PERTUSSIS)

Clinical Features

1. **C**atarrhal stage: One week. Mimics upper resp. viral infection
2. **C**ough (Spasmodic) stage: Staccato cough. Spasm followed by inspiratory whoop.
3. **C**onvalescent stage.

Complications

1. Secondary infection	Bacterial pneumonia Post-pertussis bronchiectasis Otitis media
2. Physical effects of paroxysm	
Intrathoracic	Pneumothorax Rib fracture (adults)

	Subcutaneous emphysema
	Truncal petechiae
3. Bleeding/petechiae	Epistaxis
	Facial and truncal petechiae
	Subconjunctival and scleral hemorrhage
4. Neurological	Seizures
	Encephalopathy
5. In mouth	Frenal ulcer.

DIPHTHERIA

Types

1. Respiratory:
   Faucial
   Laryngeal
   Nasal
2. Non-respiratory.

Complications

1. **Toxemia**
2. **Cardiac:** Myocarditis, cardiac arrhythmias
3. **Paralysis:**

Local:	Of palate (3rd week)
Focal:	Of accommodation (4th week)
General:	Limb weakness (5th, 6th week)
	Pharyngeal and/or diaphragmatic paralysis (7th week).

Treatment

Absolute bed rest
Antitoxin
Antibiotics (Azithromycin or erythromycin)
Airway (Tracheostomy)
Assisted respiration (if resp. paralysis).

MUMPS

Clinical Features

4 Ps

Pain beneath angle of jaw
Pyrexia
Papilla reddened
Parotid enlargement.

Complications

Common

Meningitis
Orchitis or **O**ophoritis
Pancreatitis (acute).

Rare

Mastitis
Endocardial fibrosis, encephalitis
Arthritis
Nephritis
Thyroiditis.

Differential Diagnosis of Parotid Enlargement

Local

Infection and inflammation—Suppurative parotitis, recurrent or chronic parotitis

Iatrogenic—Hypersensitivity to phenothiazines, iodide, etc.

Infiltration–by tumor

Impediment (obstruction) to major salivary ducts by calculi.

Systemic

Sarcoidosis

Sialosis

Sjögren's syndrome.

Parotid Enlargement: Bilateral

Amyloidosis

Bulimia nervosa

Cirrhosis of liver

Chronic pancreatitis

Cystic fibrosis

Parotid adenoma

Parotid cancer

Parotitis

Pituitary tumor (Growth hormone secreting)

Propylthiouracil

Sarcoidosis.

CHICKENPOX

Characteristics of Rash

CROPS
Centripetal
Rapid evolution
Oval (or elliptical)
Polymorphic
Superficial.

Complications

Acute meningitis or encephalitis
Bronchopneumonia (Widespread nodular infiltrates on X-ray)
Cellulitis
Depression of platelets (Thrombocytopenia)
Encephalopathy (allergic) or acute cerebellar
First trimester of pregnancy: Congenital abnormalities.

Unusual Forms

Bleeding (Hemorrhagic)
Bullous
Bacterial infection: Necrosis with toxemia.

Management

- Antihistamine and Lacto Calamine lotion for pruritus

- Acyclovir in adults and immunocompromised patients. Dose: 15 mg/kg 5 times a day for 7 days Given within 24 hours of symptoms
- Antibiotics for secondary infection.

MENINGITIS

Etiology

Bacterial: Meningo, pneumo, *H. influenzae, Staphylo, M. tuberculosis, Listeria monocytogenes*

Viral: Enteroviruses, polio, coxsackie, mumps, HIV, arboviruses

Genital: Herpes simplex virus types 1 and 2, other herpes viruses (cytomegalo, E-B virus, VZV), lymphocytic choriomeningitis virus

Parasitic: Amebic

Spirochetal: Syphilitic, leptospiral

Fungal: *Cryptococcus, Candida*

Aseptic:

Viral: Polio, HSV2

Partially treated pyogenic meningitis

Non-infective causes: Vasculitis (SLE), meningeal carcinomatosis, sarcoidosis, Whipple's disease

Parameningeal suppuration.

Symptoms and Signs of

(Whatever the Etiology)

1. **Infection:** Fever, rigors
2. **Irritation:** (Meningeal)

Stiffness of neck and back
Kernig's sign
Brudzinski's sign

3. **Increased intracranial pressure:**
Headache, vomiting, bradycardia, stupor or coma.

Complications

Seizures
Focal neurological deficits
Mental retardation.

TETANUS

Portals of Entry

Animal bites and stings
Burns
Compound fracture
Dental extraction
Ear piercing
Fireworks injury
Gangrenous limb
H(I)nfection: Otitis media
Iatrogenic: IM injections (e.g. quinine), unsterile or bowel surgery.

Clinical Features

Rigidity: Sardonic smile. Trismus
Reflex spasm: Spontaneous or following external stimuli

Sympathetic overaction

- **A**rrhythmias
- **BP** fluctuation
- **C**onstriction (or vasodilatation)
- **D**iaphoresis
- **E**(A)nxiety, restlessness
- **F**ever.

Types

1. Generalized
2. Clinical variants:
   - **L**ung: Local
   - **S** Splanchnic
   - **C** Cephalic
   - **A** Ascending
   - **N** Neonatal.

Main cause of death: Asphyxia, Autonomic instability.

Management

Toxin neutralization
Tranquilizers (or subtotal paralysis)
Tube (Nasogastric)
Tracheostomy
Total care (as in unconscious patient).

INFECTIOUS MONONUCLEOSIS

Clinical Features

Postcervical lymphadenopathy
Pyrexia
Pharyngeal inflammation or exudate
Palpable spleen
Palatal petechiae
Periorbital edema.

Diagnosis

WBC: Leukocytosis. 20% or more atypical lymphos.
Serology:
Non-specific: Paul Bunnel. Monospot
Specific: Anti-VCA IgG, IgM, EBV.

Complications

Antibiotic-induced skin rash
Bronchopneumonia (Interstitial pneumonitis)
Cardiac: Myocarditis. Pericarditis
Depression: (during convalescence)
Encephalitis (Also cranial nerve palsies, polyneuritis, transverse myelitis)
F(P)haryngeal edema
Glomerulonephritis
Hemophagocytic syndrome
Immunohemolytic anemia.

Rare Complications

Airways obstruction	Agranulocytosis
Arthritis	Agammaglobulinemia

VIRAL INFECTIONS

Herpes Viruses

Normal immunity		Immunocompromised	
α-herpes viruses Herpes simplex virus 1	Children Stomatitis	Adults Cold sores Keratitis Encephalitis Erythema multiforme	Dissemination
Herpes simplex virus 2	Enceph.	Primary genital herpes Recurrent gen. herpes	Dissemination
β-herpes viruses	Cytomegalo Congenital (mental retard. Hearing loss)	Infectious mononucleosis	Pneumonitis Retinitis Enteritis

Human herpes virus 6, 7	Roseola infantum Febrile fits		Encephalitis
Varicella-zoster virus	Chickenpox	Shingles: Herpetic vesicles on skin Post-herpetic neuralgia	
Human herpes virus 8		Kaposi's sarcoma Castleman dis.	
Epstein-Barr virus		Infectious mono. Kaposi's sarcoma	Lymphomas Kaposi's sarcoma Nasopharyngeal Ca. Hairy leukoplakia

Clinical Features

Arthralgia
Aplastic crises
Anemia (Transfusion-dependent)
Abortions

Viral Encephalitis

Viruses associated—

1. Arboviral
2. Unusual complication of common viral infections:
   a. Picornaviruses (polio, coxsackie, echo, entero, mumps)
   b. Adenoviruses
   c. Measles
   d. Epstein-Barr
   e. Rabies
3. Delayed onset encephalitis: Polyoma, JC-virus. Rubella and measles. Kuru and C-D (caused by prions). HIV infection
4. Herpes simplex encephalitis.

Clinical Features

Fever

Fits

Fusion (confusion), drowsiness, coma

Focal symptoms esp. in herpes simplex (anosmia, olfactory and gustatory hallucinations, memory loss, dysphasia, bizarre behavior from frontal and temporal lobe affection)

Note: These distinguish viral encephalitis from meningitis, in which there is no nervous tissue involvement.

Complications

Mental symptoms: Intellectual impairment, irritability.

Neurological: Parkinsonism, hemiparesis, deafness, ocular abnormalities.
Obesity
Polyuria
Queer involuntary movements—Choreiform, myoclonic, etc.
Respiratory disturbances: of rate and rhythm
Sleep disturbances: Lethargy, insomnia or both.

HERPES SIMPLEX INFECTIONS

Primary Infections

Anal infection (male homosexuals)
Brain invasion (Encephalitis)
Cold sores (Gingivostomatitis)
Disseminated herpes simplex
Eye infections (Keratoconjunctivitis)
Finger whitlow
Genital herpes
Herpetic rhinitis.

Recurrent Infections

Herpes labialis
Eye infections: Superficial keratitis
Genital infections—usually milder.

Complications

Encephalitis
Eczema
Erythema multiforme
Embryonic (Neonatal) infection
E(I)mmunocompromised patients (Risk of prolonged and severe recurrences).

Treatment

Specific

Valacyclovir 500 mg tds x 10 d. Contraindicated in immunocompromised
Acyclovir 400 mg tds x 10 d. Topical application for labial and genital herpes q3h.

General

- Cold compresses with tap water or Burrow's solution for 10 mts. tds when lesions are vesicular
- Cleansing mouth washes
- Corticosteroid application for recurrent lesions.

HUMAN PAPILLOMA VIRUS (HPV)

Diseases Caused

- Verrucae plantaris, palmaris
- Verrucae plena—Face, hands, forearms
- Periungual warts

- Dermal cancers—Squamous cell Ca, basal cell Ca
- Condylomata acuminata—Perianal, external or internal genitals
- Anogenital malignancies
  Cervical cancer
  Penile carcinoma
  Intraepithelial neoplasms
- Others
  Oral lesion
  Oropharyngeal cancers.

Treatment

- Verrucae
  - Keratolysis
  - Cryotherapy
- Anogenital warts
  - Podophyllum locally
  - Imiquimod 5% cream
- Ablation
  - Surgery
  - Laser
  - Electrocauterization.

POLIOMYELITIS

Factors Affecting Paralysis

Infants: Less commonly affected
Injury to muscle or hypodermic inj., tonsillectomy

Iatrogenic: Steroids (during pregnancy)
Immunosuppression.

Poliovirus Replication

Phase 1

Primary multiplication in epithelium of oropharynx, intestinal mucosa.

Phase 2

Spread of virus to regional lymph nodes and replication. Enters blood stream to produce transient viremia.

Phase 3

Virus disseminated in extraneural tissues. Extensive replication of virus here. Spread to blood stream, persistent viremia.

Clinical Features

One of the following:

1. **Inapparent infection**
2. **Abortive illness:** Flu-like illness
3. **Paralytic polio:** Constitutional symptoms followed by pain and stiffness in involved ms, followed by paralysis.

IMMUNIZATION AND VACCINATION

Toxoid Vaccines

Tetanus and diphtheria: Primary vaccination—3 doses, the first 2 doses at least 4 weeks apart and 3rd dose 6–12 months after the second. One of the doses should be Tdap (tetanus diphtheria acellular pertussis with Td (tetanus-diphtheria) for the other 2 doses.

Bacterial Vaccines

Pertussis (as above)

Meningococcus: Vaccine is given as a 0.5 mL single dose of polysaccharide vaccine subcut.

Pneumococcus: Vaccine contains purified capsular polysaccharide of 23 serotypes and is given as 0.5 mL single dose over the age of 65 or more, immunocompromised adults in adults and those with chronic illnesses like cardiovascular or pulmonary disease (excluding asthma), chronic renal disease, diabetes or alcoholism.

Typhoid fever: 3 doses of Ty21a capsules/sachets (liquid formulation) on alternate days. Booster doses once in 3 years.

Cholera: Injectable killed whole cell vaccine, 2 doses, one week to one month apart. Protection lasts for 3 months.

Inactivated Virus Vaccines

Hepatitis A

Single dose for postexposure prophylaxis (PEP) for adults aged 40 years or younger. Over age of 40, immune globulin is preferred.

Hepatitis B

2 doses at 0.1 and 6 months. When antibody levels decline to <10 mL/IU/mL, a booster dose is recommended. There is a combined HIV and hepatitis B vaccine which is administered in 3 doses at 0, 1 and 6 months.

Influenza

Vaccine contains type B and two type A strains. Single dose of the vaccine confers protection in 70–90% under age of 65 years. An intranasal preparation of live attenuated vaccine may be used for healthy non-pregnant adults <50 years of age who have no high-risk medical conditions and are not in contact of severely immunocompromised persons.

Polio

Live oral polio vaccine (OPV). Vaccinations of adults over age 18 is not recommended unless the prior series has not been completed.

Human Papilloma Virus (HPV)

Vaccine is given in 3 doses at 0.1 and 6 months for all women age 9 through 26 years of age, and ideally prior to sexual activity.

Live Virus Vaccines

Measles, Mumps, Rubella (MMR)

0.5 mL sc into deltoid. In an 0.5 mL adult with no history of vaccination, 2 doses MMR at least one month apart.

Varicella

For adults 2 doses 4–6 weeks apart. 0.5 mL sc over deltoid. It is contraindicated in pregnancy or if possibility of pregnancy within 4 weeks and in individuals with malignancy or HIV.

Pentavalent Vaccine

Protection against DPT, hepatitis B, Hib (leading cause of bacterial meningitis and second leading cause of bacterial pneumonia deaths under age of 5 years).

CHAPTER

9

Tropical Diseases

MALARIA

Clinical Features

Uncomplicated Malaria

Fever (Hot stage)
Chills (Cold stage)
Sweating stage
Myalgia, headache

Complicated Fulminant Falciparum Malaria

Anemia
Blackwater fever
Cerebral (Convulsions, drowsiness progressing to coma, hyperpyrexia, oculogyric crisis)
Distress syndrome (ARDS)
Eye (retinal) hemorrhages
Failure: Cardiac. Renal. Peripheral (shock)
Gram-negative septicemia
Hypoglycemia
Hyperlactacidemia
Intravascular hemolysis

Jaundice
P. vivax: Intermittent fever on alternate days
P. malariae: Symptoms every 72 hours.

Late Complications

Tropical splenomegaly syndrome (TSS): *P. falciparum*
Nephrotic syndrome: *P. malariae.*

Treatment

Artesunate is the most rapidly acting antimalarial drug.

KALA-AZAR

Clinical Features

Anemia
Black pigmentation
Cardiac symptoms (from severe anemia)
Diarrhea
Enlarged spleen and liver
Fever (Biphasic or double diurnal)
Generalized lymphadenopathy (esp. in children)
Hemorrhagic features (notably epistaxis).

Diagnosis

Parasitological

LD bodies in aspirate from bone marrow, spleen.

Immunological

Direct agglutination test (DAT).

Treatment

Antimonials
Aromatic diamidines (pentamidine)
Amphotericin B (liposomal)
Aminoglycoside (aminosidine)

Miltefosine.

Cutaneous Leishmaniasis

- Oriental sore. Crateriform ulcer.
- Post-kala-azar dermal leishmaniasis (PKLD)
- Erythematous nodules (periorofacial area)
- Hypopigmented macules on trunk
- Photosensitivity.

TYPHOID FEVER

Clinical Features

First Week

Insidious onset with fever, headache, malaise.

Second Week

Abdominal discomfort
Bradycardia (relative)

Coated tongue
Diarrhea
Eruption: Rose spots
Enlarged spleen
Fever: Sustained, occasionally remittent.

Third Week

Spontaneous recovery unless complications.

Complications (Mainly GI)

Abscess: Hepatic. Splenic
Bleeding (Intestinal)
Cholecystitis
Distension
Perforation
Pancreatitis
Parotitis
Peritonitis.

AMEBIASIS

Clinical Features

Intestinal amebiasis

1. Asymptomatic cyst-carriers
2. Non-dysenteric: Abdominal discomfort, constipation, flatulence

3. Dysentery
4. Fulminant necrotizing colitis (toxic megacolon).

Complications

Intestinal:	Ameboma **B**leeding **C**olitis (Post-dys.). Colonic stricture **D**icitis (Appendicitis) **E**(I)ntussusception (rare)
Hepatic:	Liver abscess
RS:	Abscess (Primary or secondary) Bronchopneumonia
CVS:	Pericarditis
Cerebral:	Brain abscess
Skin:	Perianal ulceration
Spleen:	Abscess
Urogenital:	Vaginitis Ulcer on glans penis.

Treatment

Cyst passers		Diloxanide furoate
Amebic dys	}	Metronidazole or Tinidazole or Secnidazole followed by—
Ameboma		
ALA		Diloxanide furoate

CHOLERA

Clinical Features

Stages

1. **Evacuation:** Painless, profuse diarrhea (rice water stools). Vomiting. Subnormal temperature
2. **Collapse:** Dehydration, muscle cramps. Urinary suppression. Renal tubular necrosis if prolonged hypotension
3. **Reaction:** Cessation of vomiting, less stools. Rise of BP.

Complications

Acidosis (metabolic)	Hypoglycemia
Anuria	Hypovolemic shock

Treatment

WHO oral sol.		**IV sol. (5:4:1)**	
NaCl	3.5 g	NaCl	5 g
$NaHCO_3$	2.5 g	$NaHCO_3$	4 g
KCl	1.5 g	KCI	1 g
Glucose	20 g	per liter	
per 1 L water			

Tetracycline or doxycycline.

RABIES

Transmission

Aerosol route (in bat-infected caves or lab. accidents)
Bite of rabid animal
Contamination of scratch wounds by virus laden saliva.

Clinical Features

Prodromal Stage

Personality changes (Anxiety, irritability)
Pyrexia
Pains (Headache, myalgia)
Paresthesiae at site of bite
Pruritus.

Followed By

If infection predominantly in brain:

- *Furious rabies*

  Hydrophobic spasms (ending in opisthotonus and convulsions)
  Hyperexcitability
  Hyperactivity of autonomic system
  (Salivation, sweating, tachycardia)
  Or

If infection predominantly in spinal cord:

- *Paralytic rabies (Dumb rabies):*

  Paresthesiae localized to bite site

Paralysis: begins in bitten limb (50%) and spreads rapidly and symmetrically
Hydrophobia unusual.

CHIKUNGUNYA

Transmission

Aedes aegypti.

Clinical Features

- Fever for few days
- Arthralgia. Arthritis of extremities lasting for weeks or months
- Conjunctival suffusion
- Petechiae or maculopapular rash.

Diagnosis

ELISA to detect antigen and antibody in blood.

Treatment

Symptomatic.

DENGUE

Transmission: Mosquito *Aedes aegypti.*

Clinical Features

1. **Undifferentiated fever:** In young children. Mild fever for 1–3 days.

2. **Dengue fever syndrome:**
   Acute onset with fever, retro-orbital headache, bodyache (break bone fever)
   Bleeding: GI
   Cutaneous rash: Maculopapular
3. **Dengue hemorrhagic fever (DHF):**
   Capillary leakage
   Decreased platelets
   Effusion: Pleural
   Fever: for 2 days or more
4. **Dengue shock syndrome (DSS):** Mainly in children
   - Febrile phase: Unremarkable
   - With defervescence: Sudden onset of:

Hypotension	Cold extremities
Hypovolemia	Circumoral cyanosis
Hepatomegaly	Capillary (plasma) leakage

Diagnosis

- Detection of antibodies with rising titer
- RT-PCR: Detection of virus within 1–2 days of onset.

SWINE FLU

A contagious respiratory disease caused by type A influenza virus (H1N1 strain)

Spread: Direct contact with pigs, or coughing or sneezing

Clinical features: Fever, fatigue, anorexia, sore throat. Vomiting and diarrhea
Treatment: Oseltamivir (Tamiflu) or zanamivir (Relenza).

MID EAST RESPIRATORY SYNDROME

[Mid East Respiratory syndrome corona virus (MERS-COV)].

Symptoms

1. Acute respiratory illness with fever, cough, breathlessness
2. GI symptoms including diarrhea
3. Kidney failure can occur.

Protection

1. Avoid close contact with symptoms of respiratory illness
2. Maintain hand hygiene
3. Avoid uncooked/undercooked fruits, vegetables.

EBOLA VIRUS DISEASE

Human Transmission

Director indirect contact with blood and body fluids, and possibly droplet infection.

Clinical Features

Sudden onset of fever weakness, muscle pain, headache and sore throat followed by vomiting diarrhea, rush impairment of kidney and liver function or in some cases bleeding and often fatal.

Diagnosis

ELISA/RT-PCR assays and virus isolation by cell culture.

Treatment

Symptomatic.

LATHYRISM

Stages of Neurolathyrism

1. Latent stage—Only gait is affected
2. No stick stage—Jerky steps gait
3. One stick stage—Cross-legged gait on toes due to muscle stiffness
4. Two stick stage—Slow gait with crossed legs and bending of toes
5. Crawler gait due to atrophy of lower limb muscles.

LEPROSY

Cardinal Features

1. Hypopigmented or erythematous patches

2. Thickening of peripheral nerves
3. Demonstration of AFB from skin lesions

A. **Indeterminate lesions:** Hypopigmented macules anywhere on body. 70% heal spontaneously. Confer immunity

B. **Determinate lesions:** Arise spontaneously or out of indeterminate lesions.

	Tuberculoid	**Lepromatous**
Skin		
Infiltrated lesions	Defined plaques, healing centers	Diffuse thickening
Macular lesions	Single, small	Innumerable, confluent
Peripheral n. lesions	Solitary enlarged ns.	Slow, symmetrical loss (Glove and stocking)
Immunity	++	-ve
Bacilli	Few	Plenty
Lepromin test	+ve	-ve
Antibody titer	Nil	High
Lepra reactions	Type 1—Acute inflamm. of skin lesions and affected ns.	Type 2—Erythema nodosum leprosum, or acute iritis, lymphadenitis, myositis, neuritis, or orchitis.

Dimorphous Leprosy

Borderline tuberculoid: Skin lesions more numerous and more variable in size. Peripheral nerves thickened.
Borderline lepromatous: Skin lesions less symmetrical, more easily seen. Discrete red nodules. Lesions of nose, eyes, testes, muscles and bones rare.

Drug Regimens

Types of leprosy	Regimen		Treatment duration
Pauci-bacillary	Monthly	Daily	
	Rifampicin 600 mg	Dapsone 100 mg	6 months
Multi-bacillary	Rifampicin 600 mg	Clofazimine 300 mg	24 months
	Clofazimine 300 mg	Dapsone 100 mg	
Pauci-bacillary	Rifampicin	600 mg	Single dose
	Ofloxacin	400 mg	
Single lesion	Minocycline	100 mg	

INTESTINAL WORMS

Infective Stage

Swallowed: EAT
Enterobius verm.

Penetrate skin:
Hook worm

Ascaris
Trichuris trich.
Strongyloides.

ASCARIASIS (ROUND WORM)

Clinical Features

1. Tissue (larval) phase (Lung, liver)
   Transient hepatomegaly. Pneumonitis, bronchial asthma, urticaria, Loeffler's syndrome
2. Intestinal phase:
   Passage of worms from anus or mouth
   Pain in abdomen
   Poor appetite
   Poor nutritional state.

Complications

Appendicitis
Block (obstruction): of upper resp. tract or intestine (also perforation)
Colic: Biliary, hepatic or pancreatic ascariasis.

Treatment

Mebendazole 100 mg bd x 1 day
or Albendazole 400 mg one dose
or Pyrantel 10 mg/kg one dose
or Levamisole 150 mg one dose

ANKYLOSTOMIASIS (HOOKWORM)

Clinical Features

Dermatitis on feet
Dyspnea, cough (larval phase)
Drop in Hb
Duodenal ulcer-like pains
Depraved appetite (soil eating)
Depigmentation (in dark skin)
Deterioration of general health.

Treatment

Mebendazole 100 mg bd × 3
or Albendazole 400 mg st.
or Pyrantel 10/kg od × 3.

ENTEROBIASIS (THREAD WORM)

Clinical Features

Intestinal

Anal itching and dermatitis
Appendicitis.

Non-intestinal

In young girls:
Vulvovaginitis, endometriosis, pelvic peritonitis
Enuresis.

Treatment

Mebendazole 100 mg one dose
or 10 mg/kg one dose
Repeat after 2 weeks. All family members to be treated.
Hygienic measures.

TRICHURIASIS

Clinical Features

Abdominal pain, anemia
Bloody diarrhea (and rectal prolapse) or
Constipation
Deficient growth
E(I)ntussusception.

Treatment

Mebendazole >5 years 200 mg/day x 3
<5 years 100 mg/day x 3 or
Oxantel 20 mg/kg/day x 2.

TAENIASIS

T. saginata:
Asymptomatic mostly. Occasionally straying proglottids may cause appendicitis or cholangitis.
T. solium: Cysticercosis
Brain: Convulsions. Mental disorders
Subcutaneous or muscle cysts
Other organs: Eye, liver, lung.

Treatment

Niclosamide 2 g single dose or
Praziquantel 5–10 mg/kg single dose.

STRONGYLOIDIASIS

Clinical Features

Skin Penetration

Linear eruption
Loeffler's syndrome (during lung migration)
Localized inflammation of jejunum (causing hypoproteinemia, anemia)

Acute disseminated strongyloidiasis disease may occur in:

Pregnancy
Puerperium
Prednisolone and other immunosuppressive drugs.

Treatment

Thiabendazole 25 mg/kg/day x 5 days
or Albendazole 400 mg/kg x 3 days.

GIARDIASIS

1. Asymptomatic.
2. Acute giardiasis

Anorexia
Bowel movements: Frequency with loose, foul smelling stools
Cramps: Midepigastric
Distension

3. Persistent symptomatic infection
Frequent bowel movements with soft stools
Failure to thrive in children
Folate deficiency
Flatulence
Food allergy.

Treatment (Adult)

Metronidazole 200 mg tds x 14 or 2 g single dose x 3
or Tinidazole 1.5–2 g single dose
or Furazolidone 100 mg qds x 7–10 days.

FILARIAL INFECTIONS

Main Types

- Lymphatic filariasis transmitted by mosquitoes. Can be caused by—
  Bancrofti (Wuchereria)
  Brugia malayi
  Brugia timori
- Subcutaneous fibrosis (onchocerciasis and loasis) transmitted by biting flies.

Lymphatic Filariasis

Acute

- Fever: 3–7 days. Recurring
- Adenolymphangitis:
  Funiculo-epididymo-orchitis
  Lymphadenopathy: Inguinal or axillary. Cellulitis, abscess formation.

Chronic

Hydrocele
Lymphatic rupture—Chyluria, lymphuria
Loeffler's syndrome (tropical pulmonary eosinophilia)
Lymphedema—Arm, leg, scrotum, vulva, breast (Elephantiasis).

Treatment

Diethylcarbamazine (DEC)
Ivermectin with DEC or albendazole.

PLAGUE

Types

Common

- Bubonic
- Pneumonic
- Septicemic.

Uncommon

- Cervical bubonic
- Carbuncular (at site of flea bite)
- Plague meningitis.

Complications

- Disseminated intravascular coagulation (DIC)
- Gangrene (Peripheral)
- Meningitis.

Diagnosis

WBC: Leukocytosis
Y. pestis: in material from glands, blood, sputum
Serology: Specific IgM and IgG.

Treatment

Streptomycin 15 mg/kg in two divided doses IM for 5–7 days, then Tetracycline 250–500 mg qds.
Chloramphenicol IV if meningitis and shock.

HYDATID DISEASE

Clinical Features

Asymptomatic

Especially if calcified

Of liver: All Ps
Painless hepatomegaly
Pyrexia of unknown origin
Pressure on bile ducts—Jaundice
Perforation (Rupture) giving rise to—
Systemic reaction
Rupture into pleural or peritoneal cavity, gut, biliary tree.

Lung Hydatid Cyst

Breathlessness
Bronchial ulceration—Hemoptysis
Bursting (Rupture) into bronchus—
Expectoration of daughter cysts, allergic response and resp. distress from aspiration of fluid into lung
Bacterial infection (secondary): Fever, cough, purulent sputum.

Other Sites

Neurocysticercosis

Cerebral : Seizures, syndrome of IIP, space occupying lesion syndrome, syndrome of meningoencephalitis, stroke
Spinal : Compression myelopathy, radiculopathy
Muscles : Pseudohypertrophy
Bones : Pathological fracture
Spleen : Splenomegaly

Kidneys : Hematuria
Thyroid : Goiter
Eye : Exophthalmos
Abdomen : Pseudocyesis.

Treatment

Albendazole 10–20 mg/kg/day for 4–6 weeks
Surgery if pressure symptoms or eye involvement.

BRUCELLOSIS

Clinical Features (*B. Abortus* Milder)

Acute Onset Brucellosis

Arthritis or arthralgia (with back pain)
Breathing difficulty with cough, sore throat, chest pain
Confusion (mental), nightmares
Diarrhea (or constipation), nausea, vomiting
Enlarged: Liver, spleen, lymph nodes
Funiculitis and epididymo-orchitis
Generalized aches and pains: Influenza-like illness.

Insidious Onset Brucellosis

Anorexia (and loss of weight)
Backache (with or without) joint pains
Constipation
Diaphoresis: Drenching sweats
Enlarged spleen

Fever (low grade)
Generalized aches and pains
Headache (and depression).

Diagnosis

Culture: Blood, marrow
Standard agglut. (SAG) test.

Treatment

Doxycycline 100 mg bd +
Streptomycin 1 g/day x 14 days
or Doxycycline + Rifampicin 15 mg/kg/d x 45 days
or Doxycycline 200 mg od x 6 days.

SCHISTOSOMIASIS

Clinical Features

3 Stages

1. **Skin penetration stage (Swimmer's itch)**
2. **Systemic symptoms:** Acute schistosomiasis coinciding with egg-laying by worm. Serum sickness-like syndrome
3. **Sequelae:** Complications from laying of eggs in—
   Urinary tract: Frequency, burning, dribbling. Bladder granulomas, calcification. Obstructive uropathy
   Intestines: (Colon)—Diarrhea with blood, mucus, pus
   Diffuse involvement of trans. colon

Liver and spleen: Hepatic and portal fibrosis. Splenomegaly and hypersplenism.

Pulmonary:

Arterial	– Cor pulmonale
Parenchyma	– Bronchitis, bronchiectasis, emphysema

Central Nervous System

Brain	– Tumor symptoms
Spinal cord	– Myelitis or radiculitis of cauda equina.

Diagnosis

Egg of *S. hematobium* in urine (mid day sample).
Serological tests.

Treatment

Praziquantel single oral dose of 40 mg/kg or 60 mg/kg in 3 divided doses for one day.

RICKETTSIAL DISEASES

Scrub Typhus

Transmission

Bite of larval stage of chiggers.

Clinical Features

Like common flu—
Dry cough
Eschar at site of bite
Fever

GI symptoms
Headache.

Complications

Pneumonia, myocarditis, GI bleeding, meningoencephalitis, acute kidney failure.

Diagnosis

Immunofluorescence antibody test (IFA) and indirect immunoperoxidase test.

Treatment

Doxycycline—Adult 100 mg bd, children 4 mg/kg/d x 12–14 days.

ANTHRAX

Clinical Forms

1. Cutaneous anthrax—Lesions on exposed parts. Begins as painless papule progressing to vesicles which ulcerate with a central black eschar, surrounded by a ring of vesicles. Toxic features occur in about half the cases. Healing occurs in 1–3 weeks with scarring
2. Inhalational anthrax—Used in chemical warfare
3. Gastrointestinal
4. Meningitis.

Treatment

Penicillin in large doses.

LEPTOSPIROSIS

Type	Host
L. Icterohemorrhagica	Rats and small rodents
L. grippotyphosa	Voles
L. hardjo	Cattle

Transmission

From contact with tissues of infected animal or from contaminated water or soil.

Clinical Stages

1. **Septicemic phase:** First week
   Aches and pains
   Bleeding: Petechiae, hemoptysis
   Conjunctival suffusion
   Disturbances of consciousness
   Enlarged liver, spleen
   Fever with chills
   Glandular enlargement
   Headache, often severe
   Infection: Uveitis
   Jaundice (if severe infection)
   Kidney involvement: RBCs, granular casts, kidney failure
   Lung involvement: Cough, rhonchi, crackles
2. **Immune phase:** Leptospires (only in kidney and aqueous humor)—Meningeal symptoms, rash,

secondary fever, more severe hepatic and renal manifestations (in some).

Diagnosis

Isolation of organism
Seroconversion or rise in antibody titer.

Treatment

Mild Disease

Doxycycline 100 mg po bd
Amoxycillin 500 mg po bd.

Moderate/Severe Disease

Injection Ceftriaxone 1 g/d IM or IV infusion x 7 days
Dialysis if kidney failure.

CHAPTER 10

Dermatology

TOPICAL THERAPY

Topical agent	Indications
Corticosteroids	Inflammatory dermatoses
Emollients	Xerosis, eczema, psoriasis
Retinoids	Psoriasis, acne, photodamage
Vitamin D analogues	Plaque psoriasis
Coal tar	Plaque psoriasis
Dithranol	Plaque psoriasis

TOPICAL CORTICOSTEROIDS

Potency	Corticosteroid
Mild	Hydrocortisone
Moderate	Clobetasone butyrate
Potent	Betamethasone valerate Hydrocortisone butyrate
Very potent	Clobetasol propionate

Systemic Agents

Agents/dose	Indications	Side-effects
Acitretin 0.2–1 mg/kg od	Psoriasis, ichthyoses	Mucosal dryness, myalgia, alopecia, teratogenicity, mood changes
Isotretinoin 0.5–1 mg/kg od	Acne	As above
Cyclosporin 2.5 mg/kg od	Eczema/ psoriasis	Renal impairment, infections, gum hypertrophy, hirsutism
Azathioprine 1–5 mg/kg od	Autoimmune and bullous disorders	GI symptoms, infections, myelosuppression, hepatotoxicity
Methotrexate 5–25 mg/week	Psoriasis	GI symptoms, stomatitis, myelo-suppression, liver fibrosis, nephrotoxicity.

ACNE VULGARIS

Initial lesion: Comedones—Conical raised lesion with broad base and plugged apex. Plug may be black

(black head) or white (white head). 25% white heads resolve, 75% develop into inflamed lesion.

Inflammatory lesion: Severity grades—

Grade 1 (Mild): Open and closed comedones

Grade 2 (Moderate): Comedones, papules, few pustules

Grade 3 (Severe): Predominant pustules, nodules, abscesses

Grade 4: Mainly cysts and abscesses. Widespread scarring as inflammatory lesions resolve.

Treatment

Topical therapy: Retinoids and—

Antibiotics: Erythromycin, tetracycline

Benzoyl peroxide

Combination therapies:

- Benzoyl peroxide/erythromycin
- Isotretinoin/erythromycin.

ECZEMA

Classification

Exogenous

Irritant contact dermatitis

Allergic contact dermatitis

- Photodermatitis
- Infantile dermatitis.

Endogenous

Atopic dermatitis
Seborrheic dermatitis
Nummular eczema
Asteatotic eczema
Stasis dermatitis
Pompholyx
Juvenile plantar dermatitis

- Eczema associated with systemic disease
- Eczematous drug eruption.

Treatment

Acute Eczema

Topical:
Cold compresses (15 minutes): Condy's lotion, pot. permanganate, Burrow's solution, normal saline, silver nitrate 0.5%
Local application: Corticosteroid lotion, anti-infectives, oily calamine lotion
Systemic: Antihistamines, antibacterials, corticosteroids, tranquillizers, immunosuppressives, immunomoderators (tacrolimus).

Chronic Eczema

Topical:
Corticosteroid ointment (under polythene occlusion at night) or cream, zinc oxide paste or coal tar paste.
Tacrolimus or pimecrolimus

Intralesional: Steroid injection Phototherapy (PUVA, UVR)
Systemic: Sedative antihistamine, corticosteroid, immunosuppressives, interferons.

PAPULOSQUAMOUS ERUPTIONS

Pityriasis rosea

Herald patch (Mother patch) followed after 5–15 days by widespread rash. Discrete oval lesions which form a Christmas or fir tree pattern.

Treatment

Calamine lotion or emollient cream
Topical corticosteroid if rash very pruritic.

Psoriasis

Erythematous, well-defined, dry, scaly papules and plaques of varying size, of salmon color.

Types

- Guttate
- Erythrodermic (exfoliative)
- Chronic plaque
- Pustular: Palmoplantar. Generalized
- Psoriasis unguis
- Arthropathic (including arthritis mutilans)

Regional variations: Scalp, face, eyes, body flexures, napkin area, scrotum, palms and soles.

Management

Topical
Phototherapy: UVB, UVA
Systemic
Acitretin
Cyclosporin
Hydroxyurea
Methotrexate.

Red Scaling Rashes

Causes

Psoriasis
Ringworm
Discoid eczema
Lichen simplex chronicus
Basal cell Ca (superficial)
Mycosis fungoides
Bowen's disease.

LICHEN PLANUS

Skin

- **Papulosquamous eruption**
- **Pruritus**
- **Plane topped**

- **Polyangular**
- **Purple colored**
- **Pterygium unguium and pulp tent sign**
- **Penile annular lesions.**

Mucous Membrane

1. **Oral:**
   a. Reticular: Fine lace-like network of white lines or small punctate keratoses overlying normal mucosa or
   b. Papular.
2. **Genitals:**
   a. Glans: Annular lesions appear as white striae or ulcerated plaques
   b. Vagina: Leukoplakic or erythroblastic lesions with variable atrophy.
3. **Nails:**
   Irregular longitudinal ridging of nail plate, pterygium formation, shedding of nail plate and atrophy of nail bed. Subungual hyperkeratosis.

Associated Conditions

- Autoimmune diseases: Alopecia areata, dermatomyositis
- Malignancies: Ca stomach
- Miscellaneous: UC, DM, biliary cirrhosis, chronic active hepatitis.

Treatment

Topical

Corticosteroids
Tacrolimus.

Systemic

Corticosteroids
Retinoids: Acitretin
Cyclosporin
UVA therapy.

Blistering Diseases

Inherited (Genetic)
Epidermolysis bullosa
Inflammatory
Infections: Bullous impetigo, scalded-skin syndrome
Herpes. Hand, foot and mouth disease
Insect bites
Invasion: Carcinoma, amyloidosis
Immunological: Bullous pemphigoid, pemphigus, dermatitis herpetiformis, SLE, lichen planus, porphyria cutanea tarda.
Iatrogenic: Drug reactions—
Fixed drug eruptions (e.g. barbiturates, aspirin)
Photosensitive eruptions (Phenothiazines, naproxen)
Erythema multiforme (sulfonamides, NSAIDs, anticonvulsants).

Pemphigus/Pemphigoid (e.g. penicillamine)
Toxic epidermal necrolysis (NSAIDs, sulfonamides)
Irradiation and other physical causes (e.g. irritants, heat and cold).

Treatment of Bullous Pemphigoid

1. Suppression of inflammation: Corticosteroids, antibiotics (tetracycline, sulfones) and other anti-inflammatory drugs.
2. Suppression of antibody production: High dose corticosteroid, azathioprine
3. Removal of anti-inflammatory mediators and autoantibodies: Plasmapheresis
4. Immune-modulatory therapies: IV immunoglobulin.

MOLLUSCUM CONTAGIOSUM

Cause

MC (pox) virus.

Clinical Features

Dome shaped, umbilical, waxy lesions with central punctum. Some lesions may join to form a plaque.

Distribution

In children mostly on axillae, lower abdomen, thighs and face. In adults, genital lesions usually due to sexual contact.

Resolution

In most cases spontaneous resolution over 6–9 months.

Treatment

- Cantharidin in 0.9% in flexible collodion applied on each lesion and washed off after 2–4 hours
- Application of silver nitrate 10%
- Curettage and diathermy for large lesions.

URTICARIA

Exogenous

Ingestion: Drugs (Aspirin, sulfonamides). Food, e.g. seafood
Inhalation: Pollen, plants
Irritants: Bee stings, bug bites, animal dander
Injection: Penicillin, antisera.

Endogenous

Infection: Infective hepatitis, candida infection
Infestation: Helminths, *Amoeba*
I(E)motional strain
Infiltration: Lymphomas.

Clinical Classification

1. Ordinary urticaria: Acute. Chronic
2. Physical: Cold/passive solar/dermographism

3. Contact: Immunological. Non-immunological
4. Urticarial vasculitis
5. Dermographism
6. Exercise-induced
7. Angioedema: Idiopathic. C_1 inhibitor deficiency. Drug-induced, e.g. ACEIs, aspirin.

Management

Non-Drug Therapy

Avoid aspirin, NSAIDs, Codeine, ACEIs. Overheating, alcohol

Cooling lotions

Exclusion diet.

Pharmacological Therapy

1st line	:	Antihistamine. If no response—Antagonist (H_2)
2nd line	:	Corticosteroids
3rd line	:	Immunotherapy (severe refractory auto-immune urticaria only).

Contact Urticaria

Biologic or skin contact

Due to underlying disease: Urticaria pigmentosa (mastocytoma), cutaneous vasculitis, serum sickness, malignancy.

Due to hereditary causes: Angioedema, familial cold urticaria, vibratory utricaria.

Management

1st line: Antihistamines, e.g. Doxepin.

2nd line: Systemic corticosteroids: Low dose, alternate use. Exclusion of food additives and dietary factors.

3rd line: In case of autoimmune chronic urticaria: Plasmapheresis, Cyclosporin 4 mg/kg/d x 4–6 weeks. IV immunoglobulin 2 g/kg x 5 days.

ANGIOEDEMA

Usually due to increased vascular permeability and involving deeper subcutaneous and submucosal tissues.

Classification

1. **AE with wheals:** Food (Fish, prawns). Drugs: Aspirin, NSAIDs
   Physically induced AE, angioedema eosinophilic syndrome
2. **AE without wheals (Urticaria):** Ace-inhibitor induced, hereditary
3. **Idiopathic AE.**

Management

1. Withdrawal of causative food or drugs. Injection adrenaline (1:7000) 0.2 mL SC
2. Aspirin/NSAIDs induced: Stop offending drug. Zileuton 600 mg q6–12h and Doxepin 10–25 mg q12–24h x 4 days
3. Ace-inhibitor induced: IV methylprednisolone.
4. Hereditary: Anabolic drugs, e.g. Danazol 200–600 mg or Stanozolol 1–5 mg/day.
5. Idiopathic AE: Antihistamines. Antileukotrienes (Montelukast).

MILIARIA

Types

- Miliaria rubra (Prickly heat)
- Miliaria-crystallina (Sudamina)
- Miliaria profunda
- Miliaria pustulosa.

Complications

1. Secondary bacterial infection
   Miliaria pustulosa or frank impetigo (tropical impetigo)
2. Anhidrotic asthenia if anhidrosis due to widespread *M. profunda*.

SCLERODERMA

Classification

Localized Scleroderma (Morphea)

Round or oral patches of sclerotic skin, commonest on the trunk.

Variants

Guttate

Linear/segmented

En coup de sabre: Linear sclerotic lesion, usually with childhood onset, often involves scalp or face.

Treatment

a. Topical, intralesional steroids, tacrolimus, retinoids, PUVA
b. Systemic: Hydroxychloroquine, methotrexate.

Systemic Sclerosis

Types

1. **Progressive systemic sclerosis:** Diffuse sclerosis of skin with fibrosis involving heart, lungs, GI tract, kidney. Raynaud's phenomenon is often first manifestation.
2. **CREST syndrome:** Sclerosis limited to hands and lower face may be associated with calcinosis.

Treatment

- Raynaud's: Nifedipine 10–30 mg tds, diltiazem 120–180 mg/d
- Pulse therapy with dexamethasone. Cyclophosphamide, methotrexate, immunoablation
- Stem cell therapy.

ERYTHRODERMA (EXFOLIATIVE DERMATITIS)

Etiology

1. **Pre-existing skin disease:** Atopic dermatitis, dermatophytosis, eczema.
2. **Systemic disease:** Acute or chronic leukemia, Hodgkin's, Ca lung or rectum.
3. **Drugs:** Chloroquine, gold, penicillin, dapsone, iodides, phenylbutazone.

Erythema multiforme: Target-like erythematous lesions on trunk and limbs, mucous membrane may be affected.

Stevens-Johnson syndrome: Sometimes evolves into toxic epidermal necrolysis and several drugs may trigger the condition.

Toxic epidermal necrolysis is preceded by flu-like illness followed by fever, mucous membrane involvement and extensive erythematous rash with epidermal sloughing.

	Staphylo scalded skin syndrome	Toxic epidermal necrolysis
Cause	*Staph. aureus*	Drugs, neoplasms
Age	Infants and children	Adults
Systemic symptoms	Mild	Severe
Course	1–2 weeks	>2 weeks
Prognosis	Good	Bad
Treatment	Anti-staph. drugs	Stopping offending drugs.

Drug Reactions and the Skin

Immunological

Type I hypersensitivity: Itch, urticarial rash. Less commonly bronchospasm, laryngeal edema, anaphylaxis- Aspirin, opiates, penicillins, some vaccines
Type II reactions: May produce thrombocytopenic purpura
Type III: Fever, purpuric or urticarial rash, nephritis, focal inflammation of GI tract
Type IV: Reactions to topical medications produce an eczematous reaction at site of application.

Drugs that Commonly Cause Rashes

Antibiotics (Penicillin, cephalosporins)
Anti-inflammatory drugs (NSAIDs)
Anticonvulsants
Allopurinol
Aurium (gold).

HAIR

Alopecia (Diffuse)

Causes

1. Hereditary and congenital
2. Infection: Tinea capitis, pyoderma, syphilis
3. Neoplasm
4. Systemic illness, e.g. LE
5. Telogen hair loss: Postpartum
6. Neonatal alopecia
7. Drug-induced: Antithyroid drugs, drugs affecting keratinization—Nicotinic acid, cholesterol lowering agents—Atorvastatin, rosuvastatin. Antihypertensives—Betablockers.Antiepileptics—Carbamazepine, valproate. NSAIDs, Immunomodulators—Sulfasalazine, mesalazine, immunoglobulin infusions, IFN
8. Nutritional : Protein-energy malnutrition
9. Ionizing radiation
10. Fevers: Malaria, TB, typhoid. HIV

11. Stress: Serious trauma, emotional stress, starvation
12. Malignancies: Lymphoma, leukemia
13. Organ dysfunction: Hepatic failure, kidney failure
14. Iron deficiency anemia
15. Local cause: Hair dye application.

Hirsutism

Causes

1. **Without virilization**
   Cerebral: Stress
   Pituitary: Cushing's syndrome
   Ovarian: Pregnancy, menopause
   Endocrine: Hypo- and hyperthyroidism
   Drugs: Systemic corticosteroids.
2. **With or without virilization**
   Pituitary: Hyperprolactinemia, acromegaly
   Ovarian: Polycystic ovary syndrome, theca granulosa cell tumor, metastasis, arrhenoblastoma
   Drugs: Anabolic steroid, progestins.
3. **With virilization**
   Adrenal: Congenital adrenal hyperplasia, adrenal nest tumor
   Drugs: Testosterone, synthetic androgens
   Ovarian: Ovarian hyperthecosis, hilar cell hyperplasia.

NAILS

Nail Discoloration

Yellow	Yellow nail syndrome
White	Hypoalbuminemia
Brown	Chronic kidney disease
Blue	Methotrexate, Wilson's disease
Red	Congestive heart failure
Greenish	Pseudomonas infection.

Nails in Psoriasis: SPOTS

- **S**plinter hemorrhages
- **P**itting
- **O**nycholysis
- **T**ransverse ridging
- **S**ubungual hyperkeratosis.

Longitudinal Brown Streaks in the Nails

Addison's disease
Benign racial
Carcinoma (Squamous cell)
Drugs: Minocycline, zidovudine
E(I)nfection: Fungal
Frictional
Growth: Malignant melanoma, Melanocytic nevus
Lichen planus

Koilonychia

Inherited or genetic: Nail-patella syndrome, LEOPARD syndrome, incontinentia pigmenti
Iron deficiency anemia
Injury
Skin disease: Psoriasis, lichen planus, onychomycosis, Raynaud's phenomenon
Systemic disease: Hemoglobinopathies-SG, polycythemia vera, thyroid disorders, porphyria, pellagra, malnutrition.

CUTANEOUS TUBERCULOSIS

Exogenous source	• Tuberculous chancre • Warty tuberculosis (Tuberculosis verrucosa cutis) • Lupus vulgaris
Endogenous source	
Contiguous spread	• Scrofuloderma
Auto-inoculation	• Orifacial tuberculosis
Hematogenous	• Miliary TB • Lupus vulgaris • Tuberculous gumma

Tuberculides

Micropapular	• Lichen scrofulosorum
Papular	• Papular or papulonecrotic tuberculide
Nodular	• Erythema nodosum
	• Erythema induratum

Diagnosis: Biopsy confirmatory.

PHOTOSENSITIVITY

Congenital

1. **Exaggerated sunburn response**
   - Drug-induced, e.g. thiazide diuretics, amiodarone
   - Other disorders: Xeroderma pigmentosum, erythropoietic protoporphyria.
2. **Photosensitivity induced by topical agents**
   - Phototoxicity: Concentration of photosensitizing chemical on the skin is high, so that only brief exposure to sunlight produces severe phototoxic effects including erythema, edema, blistering
   - Photoallergy, e.g. to topically applied fragrances like musk.

3. **Sun-induced blistering, e.g.**
   - Bullous porphyrias.
   - Drugs: Naproxen, nalidixic acid, fluoroquinolones.
4. **Eczema and eczema-like photosensitivity eruptions:** Photo-exacerbated seborrheic dermatitis, chronic actinic dermatitis.

Acquired

1. **Polymorphic light eruption:** Itchy, papular eruption in sun-exposed sites.
   Others: Hydroa vacciniforme, actinic prurigo, solar urticaria.
2. **Sun-aggravated disorders:** Psoriasis, eczema, erythema multiforme and herpes simplex. Also Hartnup disease, niacin deficiency (pellagra).

PIGMENTATION

Pigmented Lesions: ABCD of examination
Acquired or congenital
Border
Color
Distribution.

Hyperpigmentation

Localized

- Cafe au lait spots
- Freckles

- Melasma (Pregnancy mask)
- Melanoma
- Melanocytic nevus
- Fixed drug eruption
- Benign nevus.

Generalized

- Addison's disease
- Acanthosis nigricans
- Biliary cirrhosis
- Hemochromatosis
- Vitamin B_{12} deficiency
- Chronic kidney failure
- Glycogen storage disease
- Gaucher's disease.

Hypopigmentation

Localized

Leprosy
Vitiligo
Pityriasis alba
Pityriasis versicolor
Tuberous sclerosis
Post-inflammatory
Nevus anemicus.

DERMATOSES OF PREGNANCY 4 PS

Polymorphic eruption of pregnancy
Itchy papules in striae

Prurigo of pregnancy
Itchy papules on abdomen and limbs

Pemphigoid gestationis
Urticated erythema, bullae, often periumbilical

Pruritic folliculitis
Itchy, follicular papules.

CHAPTER 11

Sexually Transmitted Infections

BACTERIAL INFECTIONS

Syphilis

1. Congenital
   - Early
   - Late (stigmas)
2. Acquired
   - Early.

Primary

Sore or chancer at site of entry of organism, with regional lymphadenitis.

Secondary

1. Rash: Usually nonpruritic. Papular syphilide earliest and most common. Variants–follicular, annular, corymbose. Papules: Condylomata lata in warm moist areas.
2. Lymphadenopathy.
3. Mucosal lesions: Mucous patches, snail-track ulcers.

- Early latent
- Late: Late latent
  Tertiary (Gummatous)
  Quaternary (CVS or Neuro).

Gonorrhea

- Gonococcal urethritis in men
- Genital gonorrhea in women
- Rectal gonorrhea
- Vulvovaginitis in children
- Ophthalmia neonatorum.

Disseminated gonococcal infection: Skin, arthritis, endocarditis and meningitis.

Chancroid (Soft Sore)

Organism: *H. ducreyi.*
Clinical features: Papule. Papulopustule, Ulcer: Ulcers usually superficial, painful, ragged., floor covered by exudate.
Site: *Male:* Prepuce, coronal sulcus, ext. urinary meatus. *Female:* Fourchette, vestibule, labia minora, perianal region.
Variations: Transient (bubo), dwarf, giant, phagedenic, papular, serpiginous, granulomatous (resembling granuloma inguinale).

Lymphogranuloma Venereum

Organism: *Klebsiella trachomatis.*

Primary stage: Herpetiform—Superficial, painless, evanescent lesion. No scar. Less commonly ulcer, papule or nodule.

Inguinal syndrome: Enlargement of inguinal lymphnodes above and femoral nodes below. Poupart's ligament creates a groove between the two (sign of groove). Fever, chills, arthralgia.

Genito-anorectal syndrome: Genitals in both sexes undergo hyperplasia. Edema of rectal mucosa. Multiple fissures radiating from anal margin. Rectal strictures.

Granuloma Inguinale (Donovanosis)

Organism: *Klebsiella granulomatis.*

Early lesion: Papule firm. In few days, overlying epithelium exfoliates to form bright pink painless ulcer which bleeds to touch. In both sexes, disease spreads to or occurs in inguinal and perianal regions. In some there is subcut. swelling in inguinal region (pseudobubo) which bursts to produce ulcer.

Fully developed lesion:

1. Hypertrophic verrucous type
2. Sclerotic or cicatricial type
3. Fleshy exuberant type
4. Necrotic type.

Bacterial Vaginosis

Protozoal and Fungal Infections

Trichomoniasis
Genital candidiasis
Vaginal infection
Balanitis/Balanoposthitis.

Crab Lice and Scabies

Non-specific genital infection (NSGI)
Nonspecific urethritis (NSU).

Viral Infections

- Genital herpes
- Genital warts and genital papilloma virus disease
- Molluscum contagiosum
- Viral hepatitis B (HBV)
- HIV.

HIV AND AIDS

Transmission

1. Sexual
2. Blood and tissue fluids
3. Contaminated needles and syringes
4. Organ and tissue donation
5. Mother to child during birth process.

Stages of HIV Infection

1. Primary infection/Acute HIV syndrome.
   Seroconversion illness with fever, skin rash, myalgia, fall in CD4 count. Spontaneous recovery in few weeks in majority.
2. Early immune deficiency: CD4 >500/μL
   Usually asymptomatic but viral replication continues.
3. Intermediate immune deficiency (CD4 200–500)
   Compromised immune system. Subtle clinical features.
4. Advanced immune deficiency: CD4 <200. Pt highly immunosuppressed. Major opportunistic infections and malignancies develop.

Laboratory Classification of HIV

Absolute CD4 count	Cl. category		
1. ≥500	A	B	C
2. 200–499	A1	B1	C1
3. <200	A2	B2	C2

A–Asymptomatic disease
B–Symptomatic disease mainly dermatological
C–AIDS and cutaneous.

Clinical Manifestations of HIV

Primary HIV Infection

Asymptomatic or "glandular fever-like illness". Meningoencephalitis illness and peripheral neuropathy. Usually self-limiting.

Early Manifestations

Asymptomatic or enlarged lymph nodes with or without minor symptoms. Bacterial sepsis in form of pneumonia or bacteremia.

Late Manifestations

- Constitutional symptoms and/or diarrhea, fever for >one month or wt. loss
- Neuropathic myelopathy
- Recurrent Salmonella bacteremia, extensive herpes zoster, oral candidiasis and oral hairy leukoplakia.

Opportunistic Infections in HIV

CD4 <500: TB, herpes zoster, Candida albicans
CD4 <200: Pneumocystis jiroveci pneumonia
CD4 <100: Toxoplasmosis, cryptococcus, CMV infection
Tuberculosis is the earliest HIV related OI. It is the only transmissible OI.

Complications

Cardiac Complications
Pericardial effusion, arrhythmias, heart muscle disease. Rarely pulmonary hypertension.
Neurological

1. Meningitis (TB, *Cryptococcus neoformans*).

2. Non-focal brain involvement. AIDS dementia complex, encephalopathies, progressive multifocal leukoencephalopathy, primary CNS lymphomas.
3. Focal CNS disease—Cerebral toxoplasmosis.

Spinal cord lesions: TB and pyogenic infections, CMV, peripheral neuropathies, myopathies.

Gastrointestinal Tract

1. Oral candidiasis, gingivitis, stomatitis, herpes simplex, CMV infection, hairy leukoplakia, Kaposi's sarcoma, oral warts
2. Esophageal candidiasis, ulcers, esophagitis
3. Diarrhea.

Infections

Bacterial, protozoal, Hepatitis D, pancreatitis.

Dermatological

Infections—Fungal, mycobacterial, viral. Papulosquamous disorders like psoriasis, lichen planus, Reiter's syndrome.

Malignancies

Kaposi's sarcoma, basal cell Ca, malignant melanoma.

Hematological

Neutropenia, thrombocytopenia.

Rheumatological

1. Due to impaired immunity—Infective arthritis.
2. Due to host response to HIV—Polymyositis, vasculitides.

3. Due to persistence of antigen–Reiter's syn., psoriatic arthropathy.

Cancer

Kaposi's sarcoma, non-Hodgkin lymphoma, primary cerebral lymphoma, cervical carcinoma.

Antiretroviral Therapy (ART)

Drugs

NRTIs
NNRTIS
PIs

Time of Initiation of ART

CD4 count <200	Start ART
CD4 count <350	Defer
CD4 between 200–350	Offer ART
Plasma viral load >5,00,000/mL	Start
If OIs	Defer ART until tr. of OI completed or pt. stabilized, then start
Plasma HIV RNA levels >3,000 copies/mL irrespective of $CD4^+$ T cell count and CD4 + T counts <350/mL irrespective of RNA levels.	Therapy recommended

CHAPTER

12

Psychiatry

MOOD DISORDERS

Depression

Symptoms

General

Low mood
Low self-esteem
Loss of interest
Low energy
Hopelessness
Helplessness
Pessimism
Poor concentration
Depersonalization

Somatic

Appetite disturbance
Amenorrhea
Body weight change
Constipation
Disturbance of sleep.

Treatment

Antidepressants.

ECT

Psychological treatments.

Anxiety

Tension

Apprehension

Phobias.

Features of Anxiety

Psychological: Fear +

Inner tension (and restlessness)

Irritability

Impaired ability to concentrate

Increased startle response

Increased sensitivity to physical sensations

Impaired sleep.

Physical

Dry mouth

Difficulty swallowing

Dizziness

Diarrhea

Discomfort in chest.

Tremor

Sweating

Frequency of micturition

Panic Disorders

Panic attack (acute intense anxiety attack)
Sudden onset
Short duration
Symptoms of breathlessness and/or palpitations
Shifting quickly from situation where attack occurred
Fear of impending doom.

Phobic Disorders

Specific Phobias

Single, discrete fears of an object, circumstance or situation.

Agoraphobia

Fear of crowded places where escape may be difficult. Often associated with panic disorder.

Social Phobia

Fear of being evaluated or criticized by others.

Obsessive Compulsive Neurosis (OCN)

Symptoms can arise acutely or insidiously .

Obsessions

Frequent and persistent thoughts, impulses or images normally experienced as senseless, e.g. contamination, sexual or religious ruminations.

Compulsions

Repetitive behaviors, e.g. hand washing, ordering or mental acts (e.g. counting, repeating words silently).

Management

1. Cognitive behavior therapy
2. Pharmacotherapy: SSRIs
3. Psychosurgery for Pts with severe illness not responding to multiple therapeutic approaches.

EATING DISORDERS

Anorexia Nervosa

Weight loss primary feature.

Restricting Type

Weight loss by eating restriction alone.

Binge-eating/Purging Type

Caloric restriction with other means of weight control—self-induced vomiting and abuse of laxatives.

Complications

GI

Dental erosion	*Hematological*
Parotid enlargement	Neutropenia

Esophagitis
Mallory-Weiss tear
Pancreatitis
Constipation

CVS

Arrhythmia
Bradycardia
Cardiac failure on refeeding
Decreased BP
ECG changes

Metabolic-Nutritional

Metabolic acidosis
Hypokalemia
Hyponatremia
Hypocalcemia

Anemia
Thrombocytopenia

Endocrine

Amenorrhea
Low testosterone
High cortisol

Musculoskeletal

Osteoporosis
Proximal myopathy

Skin

Lanugo hair, dry skin

Hypercarotenemia
Zinc deficiency
Thiamine deficiency
Refeeding edema

Bulimia Nervosa

Binge acting with a sense of loss of control.

Complications

Hypokalemia
Metabolic alkalosis
Dental erosion
Parotid enlargement
Hyperamylasemia
Mallory-Weiss tear

SCHIZOPHRENIA

Clinical Features 4As

Ambivalence: Inability to decide for or against
Autism: Withdrawal into self.
Affect disturbance, e.g. inappropriate action
Association disturbances: Loosening of association, thought disorder.

Clinical Presentation

Acute Schizophrenia

Delusions
Hallucinations
Thought disorder
Catatonic phenomena (e.g. mutism, stupor, strange postures or movements)
Mood changes. Perplexity or blunted effect or incongruity of mood.

Chronic Schizophrenia

'Negative' symptoms such as lack of initiative or drive, poverty of speech, social withdrawal, emotional blunting.

Treatment

Antipsychotics
Psychological
Social support, counseling.

ORGANIC AND SYMPTOMATIC MENTAL DISORDERS

Confusion

May be a symptom of:

- Recent physical trauma or head injury
- Liver disease
- Kidney disease
- CNS or systemic infection
- Endocrine disease: DM, hyper- or hypothyroidism,
- Cushing's disease, Addison's disease
- Asphyxia due to cardiorespiratory disease.

Delirium

Causes

Infection : CNS, pneumonia, typhoid fever
Injury : Post-concussional
Infiltration : Brain tumor
Infarct : Cerebral. Also SAH
Insufficiency : Hepatic or kidney failure
Iatrogenic : Drug ingestion, drug withdrawal
Endocrine : Hyper- or hypothyroidism.

Diagnosis

Impairment of consciousness and attention
Illusions and hallucinations (most often visual)
Increased reaction time and startle reaction
Insomnia. Disturbing dreams and nightmares
I (E)motional disturbances: Depression, anxiety, agitation.

Dementia

Features

Chronic brain disorder with progressive impairment of intellectual functions, behavior and personality.

Causes

Alzheimer's disease and other cerebral degenerations, e.g. Huntington's, J-C disease
Blood vessel disease: Multiple infarcts (MID)
Chronic alcoholism
Deficiency disease: Pellagra
Endocrine (and metabolic): Hypothyroidism, hypoglycemia, uremia, liver failure
Fracture skull (Head injury)
Growths (Intracranial)
Hydrocephalus (Normal pressure)
Infections: Encephalitis.

Alzheimer's Disease

Pathogenesis

Plaques
Tangles.

Diagnostic Criteria

Age: 40–90 years
Behavioral changes

Consciousness disturbed
Disturbances of language and visual skills
Episodic memory impairment
Family history of Alzheimer's disease
Gradual decline in ADL resulting in severe disability and dependance on others.

SUBSTANCE USE DISORDERS

Alcohol (Refer page 422)

Opioid Derivatives

Example: morphine, codeine, heroin, pethidine, etc.

Acute Intoxication

Apathy
Bradycardia
Constricted pupils
Depression of respiration
Excitation (initial brief)
Fall in BP.

Withdrawal Symptoms

Anxiety (severe)
Bodyache
Cramps in muscles
Dilated pupils

E(I)nsomnia
Fever
GI symptoms
Hypertension (mild)
Increased lacrimal and nasal secretions.

Cannabis

Hashish, ganga, bhang. Active ingredients labeled marijuana.

Physical Dependence

Mild.

Withdrawal Symptoms

Mild (fine tremors, irritability, restlessness, insomnia, decreased appetite).

Psychological Dependence

Varies from mild (occasional 'trips') to compulsive state.

TREATMENT METHODS IN PSYCHIATRY

Antipsychotic Drugs

Antipsychotic	Dose (mg/day po)
Typical	
Chlorpromazine	25–100
Thioridazine	150–800

Trifluoperazine	10–50
Haloperidol	15–120
Droperidol	20–120
Flupenthixol	6–18
Sulpiride	400–2400
Pimozide	2–20
Atypical	
Clozapine	25–900
Olanzapine	5–20
Quetiapine	150–750
Risperidone	2–16
Ziprasidone	20–240
Aripiprazole	5–30

Psychotherapies

Psychotherapy is an effective primary treatment for psychiatric disorders, namely—phobias, depression, post-traumatic stress disorder, borderline personality disorders, anorexia nervosa. And combined with other forms of treatment, it is a vital part of management of obsessive-compulsive disorder, substance use, schizophrenia.

Psychoanalytical psychotherapy for patients with borderline personality disorder or relationship difficulties or some psychosexual disorders.

Cognitive

Behavior therapy: Formulation based on 'ABC' principle of—
Antecedents
Behavior
Consequences.

Indications

Depression (particularly long-standing), anxiety/panic disorder, chronic fatigue syndrome, bulimia nervosa, OCD, schizophrenia.

Systemic (Family/Marital) Therapies

Integrative Therapies

Because patients often have a range of different problems (e.g. agoraphobia and marital difficulties), it can be helpful to combine or integrate therapeutic strategies.

Electroconvulsive Therapy (ECT)

Indications

- Major depression not responding to antidepressant drugs:
  With psychotic symptoms
  With failure to eat and drink
  With depressive stupor

With high risk of suicide
- Schizophrenia (especially with positive symptoms)
- Mania not responding to drug treatment
- Postpartum psychosis
- Severe catatonia.

Contraindications

Absolute: Raised intracranial pressure
Relative: Recent MI, severe hypertension, CVA, severe lung disease, detachment of retina.

rTMS therapy using magnetic field externally to stimulate nerve cells in the brain at a predetermined site on the scalp.

Advantage—Quick onset of therapeutic effect. No anesthesia.

SEXUAL PROBLEMS

Sexual Dysfunction

Male Problems

Loss of Libido

Common causes:
- Marital conflict
- Alcohol abuse
- Physical illness
- Depression
- Work stress
- Tiredness.

Erectile Dysfunction

Causes

Organic

Vascular disease (in middle aged or elderly)

Neuropathy: Diabetes, multiple sclerosis

Nerve damage: Injury or pelvic surgery

Local penile deformities

Drugs and toxins: β-blockers, certain antidepressants, anticonvulsants, H_2-receptor blockers. Tobacco. Alcohol.

Psychological factors such as performance anxiety.

Premature ejaculation due to lack of ejaculatory control.

Retarded or absent ejaculation may be due to organic or psychological or emotional factors.

Female Problems

Loss of Libido

Causes:

- Marital conflict
- Undiagnosed depression
- Tiredness from demands of employment and children, psychological adjustment to gynecological surgery.

Vaginismus

Primary: Negative or strict upbringing about sex, or sexual abuse as a child.

Secondary: Sexual assault, clumsy medical vaginal examination, painful vaginal infection, complications of episiotomy.

Other causes: Insufficient vaginal lubrication, insufficient foreplay, or side-effect of a drug, e.g. β-blockers.

Anorgasmia

Primary due to lack of foreplay, secondary from conflict within a relationship, or pelvic surgery.

Gender Disorders

Cross-Dressing

Men dressing in female garments to enhance their sexual arousal. Other men feel a compulsion to dress as a female, and describe a sense of relaxation and well-being when they do so (transvestism).

Transsexuality

Some individuals feel so unhappy with the gender of their birth and so much in 'sympathy' with the opposite sex gender that they seek full gender reassignment, hoping they will be happy in their new sex.

PERINATAL PSYCHIATRY

Common psychological symptoms following childbirth:

- Anxiety
- Altered mood
- Ambivalence about the baby

- Absent or reduced sexual interest
- Anger and bitterness
- Altered energy (inadequacy).

CHILDHOOD PSYCHIATRY

Behavioral Disorders of Children

Conduct Disorders

Repetitive antisocial behavior, defiance, hostility in young children; stealing, truancy, lying in older children.

Hyperkinetic Disorders

- Attention deficit
- Hyperactivity
- Impulsivity.

Mixed Disorders of Conduction and Emotions

Mixture of emotions and behavioral problems.

Mental Retardation

Causes

Inherited: Down's, fragile X, phenylketonuria
Infections: CMV, rubella, measles, AIDS
Injury in childhood
Idiopathic (No identifiable cause).

Diagnostic Criteria

Impaired adaptive behavior
Intellectual disability as determined by IQ
Increased prevalence of epilepsy, psychiatric disorders, hearing and visual impairment.

Autism

Diagnostic criteria

- Qualitative impairment in social interaction
- Qualitative impairment in verbal and nonverbal communication
- Restrictive, repetitive and stereotyped patterns of behavior, interests and activities.

CHAPTER

13

Pediatrics

RESUSCITATION OF THE NEWBORN

TABCs of resuscitation

T Temperature maintenance
- Radiant heat source
- Skin-to-skin contact with the mother
- Removing wet linen

A Airway
- Position infant
- Suction of mouth, nose, if necessary trachea

B Breathing initiation
- Tactile stimulation to initiate respiration
- PPV if necessary (with bag, or bag and ET tube)

C Circulation
- Stimulation and maintenance with chest compressions and/or medications.

NEONATAL JAUNDICE

Physiological

- Increased bilirubin load on liver cells
- Defective hepatic uptake of bilirubin
- Defective bilirubin conjugation
- Defective bilirubin excretion.

Pathological (Unconjugated Bilirubin)

Increased Production

Incompatibility: Rh, ABO
Inherited: Hereditary spherocytosis
Infection
Increased enterohepatic circulation: Pyloric stenosis
Non-spherocytic hemolytic anemia.

Decreased Clearance

Inborn error of metabolism: Crigler-Najjar syndrome
Insufficiency (Thyroid).

Complications

Transient encephalopathy
Kernicterus, Phases:
I: Lethargy, poor suck, hypotonia
II: Fever, opisthotonus
III: High-pitched cry, convulsions, death.

Treatment

Exchange transfusion
Phototherapy.

HEMORRHAGIC DISEASE OF NEWBORN

Causes

Anoxia (Asphyxia)
Birth injury
Congenital thrombocytopenia
Deficient factors of coagulation
E (I) infection: Septicemia, umbilical sepsis.

LOW BIRTH WEIGHT (LBW) BABIES

Preterm

Problems

Apneic spells. Acidosis (metabolic)
Birth asphyxia
Circulatory: Intraventricular hemorrhage
Distress (Respiratory)
Enterocolitis (necrotizing)
Feeding difficulties
Gastroenteritis
Hyperbilirubinemia
Infections.

Small for Gestational Age

Problems

Asphyxia
Congenital malformation
Polycythemia
Hypoglycemia
Hypothermia
Immune status: Low
Intelligence: Poor
Persistent fetal circulation
Postnatal growth retarded.

INFANTILE CONVULSIONS

Causes

Asphyxia at birth
Brain lesion: Encephalopathy (hypertensive, post infectious)
Circulatory: A-V malformation, intracranial hemorrhage or thrombosis
Drugs (and toxins): Phenothiazines, salicylates
Epilepsy
Febrile convulsions
Growths: Tuberculoma, cysticercosis
Hypocalcemia, hypomagnesemia, dyselectrolytemia
Infection: Meningitis, encephalitis, septicemia.

FAILURE TO THRIVE

Causes

1. Non-organic/psychosocial/environmental
   Poverty
   Poor mother child relationship, psychological disturbed mother
   Poor feeding technique
2. Organic causes
   Inadequate food intake
   Inability to assimilate
   Inability to utilize
   Inborn errors causing retarded growth
   Increased metabolism.

PROTEIN-ENERGY MALNUTRITION

Clinical Features of Kwashiorkor and Marasmus

	Kwashiorkor	Marasmus
Wasting	Little	Severe
Edema	Yes	No
Subcut. fat	Present	Minimal
Muscle wasting	Variable	Severe
Serum albumin	Low	Near normal
	Enlarged, fatty liver	
	High prevalence of infection	

ACUTE DIARRHEA

Causative Agents

Infections

- **Viruses:** Rotavirus, Norwalk agent, Adenovirus, Calicivirus, Arbovirus, Enteroviruses.
- **Bacteria:** *E. coli, Shigella, Salmonella, Campylobacter jejuni, Staph. aureus, Vibrio cholerae*
- ***Yersinia enterocolitica***
- **Protozoa:** *E. histolytica, Giardia*
- **Helminths:** *Strongyloides stercoralis, Trichuris trichiura*
- **Fungal:** *Candida albicans, Cryptosporidium*
  Associated with urinary and respiratory infections.

Non-infections

- Food allergy
- Drug-induced, e.g. amoxycillin
- Emotional
- Dietetic: Overfeeding of fats, carbohydrates.

DEHYDRATION

Assessment

	Mild	Moderate	Severe
GC	Normal	Restless	Lethargic, drowsy
Eyes	Normal	Sunken	Very sunken, dry
Tongue	Moist	Dry	Very dry
Tears	Present	Reduced	Absent
Thirst	Normal	Thirsty	Drinks poorly or unable to drink

WHEEZING

Common Causes

Asthma
Acute bronchitis, bronchiolitis
Aspiration
Adenopathy: Tuberculous, mediastinal.

CHAPTER 14

Miscellaneous

RHEUMATOLOGY

Arthritis

Classification

Romantic House Surgeon

Rheumatic fever
Rheumatoid arthritis
Osteoarthritis
Metabolic: Gout
Allergic (Serum sickness)
Neuropathic (Charcot's joint)
Tuberculous
Injury
Connective tissue diseases

Clutton's:	Symmetrical
	Syphilitic
	Synovitis
House:	Hematological: **Hemophilia**
	Hemoglobinopathies
Surgeon:	Septic

Acute Polyarthritis

With Predominant Joint Diseases

RA (acute onset)
Rheumatic fever
Reiter's syndrome
Gonococcal arthritis
Gout (and pseudogout).

With Predominant Systemic Disease

SLE
Still's disease
Sarcoidosis (with erythema nodosum)
Seronegative arthritis, e.g. psoriatic arthritis
System (multi) disorder: PAN, SLE.

RHEUMATOID ARTHRITIS

Diagnostic Criteria

1. Arthritis of 3 or more joints
2. Arthritis of hand joints (wrist, metacarpal)
3. Symmetrical arthritis
4. Rheumatoid nodules
5. Serum rheumatoid factor
6. Radiographic features of RA: NOSE
   Narrowing (uniform) of joint spaces
   Osteoporosis (juxta-articular)
   Soft tissue changes
   Erosions at margins of joints.

Extra-articular Features of RA

Common

Anemia
Bursitis (and tendinitis)
Carpal tunnel syndrome
Depression
Episcleritis
Fever
Lymphadenopathy
Leg ulcers
Muscle wasting
Nodules
Nail fold vasculitis
Osteoporosis
Peripheral neuropathy.

Uncommon

Pleural effusion
Pulmonary fibrosis
Pericarditis
Systemic vasculitis.

Management

Avoidance of—Cold, dampness
Bed rest—if fever or rapid progress
Correction of—Anemia, focal infection.

Drugs

- **NSAIDs**

Drug	*Dose*
Ibuprofen	400–600 mg 1–1–1
Ketoprofen	50 mg 2–2–2
Naproxen	500 mg bd
Aceclofenac	100 mg 1–0–1
Piroxicam	20 mg od
Indomethacin	25 mg tds
Etoricoxib	60–120 mg
Etodolac	300 mg bd

- **DMARDs**

Sulfasalazine	500 mg/day increased to 1 g/d
Hydroxychloroquine	50 mg bd till response, then 200 mg od
D-penicillamine	125 mg at night increased to max. 1500 mg
Gold	
Oral	3 mg bd
IM	20–50 mg/week

- **Cytotoxic agents**

Methotrexate	7.5 mg weekly increased to 15–20 mg
Azathioprine	25 mg/kg/d
Leflunomide	100 mg od x 3 days then 20 mg od

- **Immunosuppressant**

- **Biological response modifiers:**
  Infliximab — 5 mg/kg IV at 0,2, 6 weeks and every week thereafter
- **Corticosteroids**
  Oral prednisolone — 7.5 mg/d
  Intra-articular into inflamed joints
  Oral pulse or IM or IV during flare up

Extra Measures

Splinting

Special aids and appliances

Surgery: Synovectomy, arthroplasty.

SERONEGATIVE POLYARTHRITIDES

Common Features

Peripheral inflammatory arthropathy plus

Absence of rheumatoid factor

B27-(HLA) association common

C(S)acroiliitis

Demonstration of clinical overlap between members of the group

Enthesopathy (Pathological changes at sites of insertion of ligaments or tendons)

Familial aggregation.

SERONEGATIVE ARTHRITIDES

1. **Ankylosing spondylitis**
   Clinical criteria:
   Limited movement of lumbar spine
   Lumbar spine (or dorsolumbar junction) pain
   Limited chest expansion (<2.5 cm)
   In advanced cases, thoracic kyphosis, hyperextension of neck and loss of lumbar spine movements
   Radiological: Unilateral sacroiliitis grade III-IV or bilateral sacroiliitis grade II
2. **Psoriatic arthritis**
   Distal interphalangeal joint dis. (DIP)
   Arthritis mutilans
   Peripheral oligoarthritis or polyarthritis
   Spondylitis
3. **SAPHO** (Synovitis, acne, pustulosis, hyperostosis of the spine and osteitis)
   Arthritis particularly of sternoclavicular and acromioclavicular joints
4. **Enteropathic arthritis**
   Peripheral oligoarthritis associated with inflammatory bowel disease
   Spondyloarthritis with sacroiliitis.

OSTEOARTHRITIS

1. **Primary:** No apparent cause
2. **Secondary:**
   Avascular necrosis
   Black urine (Ochronosis)
   Congenital dislocation of hip
   Dysplasia of joint
   Endocrine: Acromegaly
   Fracture dislocation of joint
   Previous joint: Surgery, inflammation, radiation
   Perthes disease.

Osteoarthritis 'Subsets'

- **Nodal generalized**: (Heberden's, Bouchard's nodes)
  Predominance in females
  Peak onset in middle age (menopause)
  Prevalence in families
  Predisposition to later osteoarthritis of knee, hip, spine
- **Large joint osteoarthritis**: Hip, knee. Usually bilaterally symmetrical.

Management

Non-surgical Treatment

Pharmacological

- Analgesics and anti-inflammatory drugs
- Intra-articular corticosteroids
- Glucosamine sulfate and/or chondroitin.

Non-pharmacological

- Weight reduction
- Physiotherapy and occupational therapy
- Aids (e.g. shoe wedges, patella-taping, stick).

GOUT

Urate Gout

Stages

1. **Hyperuricemia—Causes:**

   Decreased excretion of uric acid:

   Primary: Idiopathic. Familial juvenile gouty nephropathy

   Secondary

   Acidosis (Lactic)—Exercise, starvation, vomiting.

   Blue line on gums (Lead poisoning)

   Congenital: Down's syndrome

   Drugs: Diuretics, low dose salicylates, pyrazinamide, ethambutol, nicotinic acid, cyclosporin

   Ethanol consumption

   Failure: Chronic kidney failure.

   Increased production of uric acid:

   Primary: Increased purine synthesis *de novo*

   - Idiopathic
   - Hypoxanthine-guanine phosphoribosyl transferase deficiency

Secondary: Increased purine synthesis *de novo* following increased catabolism of purine nucleotides

- G-6-P-D deficiency (Glycogen storage disease type I)
- Myogenic (Glycogen storage disease type III, V, VII)
- Hereditary fructose intolerance.

Increased turnover of preformed purines

- Lymphoproliferative and myeloproliferative disorders: Hodgkin's, leukemia, myeloma, polycythemia vera, Waldenstrom's macroglobulinemia
    - Cytotoxic drugs
    - Carcinomatosis
    - Secondary polycythemia
    - Severe exfoliative psoriasis.

Precipitating factors of urate gout:

Alcohol excess
Bulimia (Dietary excess)
Constitutional illness
Drugs: Diuretics, allopurinol, B_{12}
Exercise (excessive)
Fasting (severe dieting)
Trauma
Surgery.

2. **Acute arthritis:** Big toe. Less often metatarsal joints, ankle, knee. Resolve in 3–10 days followed by asymptomatic period of variable duration.
3. **Intercritical period:** Attacks more severe, longer in duration, often involve additional joints.
4. **Chronic tophaceous gout:** Deposits of monosodium urate subcutaneous (most commonly on extensor surfaces of elbows or at sites of minor trauma). Intra-articular and periarticular deposits results in end-stage degenerative arthritis.

Calcium Pyrophosphate Gout ('Pseudogout')

Primary: AD inheritance
Secondary:

Hyperparathyroidism	Hypothyroidism
Hemochromatosis	Hypophosphatasia
Hypomagnesemia	Hemosiderosis

Acute mono or oligoarthritis of knee, wrist or ankle.

X-ray: Of knee shows chondrocalcinosis (Linear calcification within articular cartilage or menisci).
Synovial fluid: Rhomboid crystals.

Apatite Gout

Calcific periarthritis and tendinitis of shoulders and hips commonly. X-ray: Well defined, periarticular, cloud-like calcification.

Neuropathic Arthritis

Causes: DISTIL

Diabetes mellitus

Intra-articular injection (Steroids)

Syringomyelia (and other spinal cord lesions)

Tabes dorsalis

Indifference to pain (Congenital)

Leprosy (and other polyneuropathies).

Oligoarthritis

Gout

Reactive arthritis/Reiter's

Osteoarthritis

Psoriatic arthritis

Early RA.

Symmetrical Polyarthritis

RA

SLE

Psoriatic arthritis

Polyarticular gout

Post-infective arthritis.

ACUTE RHEUMATIC FEVER

Criteria for Diagnosis

Major Criteria

Carditis	Carditis
Can	Chorea
Produce	Polyarthritis
Numerous	Nodules (subcutaneous)
Extrasystoles	Erythema marginatum.

Minor Criteria 4 Ps

Pyrexia
Polyarthralgia
Prolonged PR interval
Persistently elevated inflammatory markers.

Diagnosis requires 2 major or 1 major and 2 minor criteria, evidence of recent streptococcal infection.

Management

Strict bed rest
Streptococcal elimination (with antibiotics)
Salicylates
Steroids.

REITER'S SYNDROME

Clinical Features

- History of GI or genitourinary tract infection within last 6 weeks
- Systemic symptoms: Fever, malaise
- Lower limb oligoarthritis of knee, ankle and/or metatarsal joints
- Enthesitis at tendo Achilles and plantar fascia insertions at calcaneum
- Tenosynovitis, often at toes, produces dactylitis or 'sausage toes'
- Acute sacroiliitis
- Skin and MM lesions (Psoriasis form)
- Gut inflammation of both small and large intestines
- Red eyes may occur.

LYMPHADENOPATHY

Causes

1. **Inflammatory or infective**
   ACUTE:
   Local: Streptococcal, lymphogranuloma inguinale, tularemia, filaria.
   Systemic illness: Rubella, infectious mononucleosis, acute viral hepatitis.

CHRONIC:
Bacterial: TB
Viral: HIV, Epstein-Barr
Protozoal: Brucellosis, toxoplasmosis, leishmaniasis.
Fungal: Histoplasmosis, coccidioidomycosis

2. **Reticuloses and blood diseases**
   Lymphocytic leukemia
   Lymphomas
   Sarcoidosis
   Toxoplasmosis
3. **Neoplasms (secondary Ca)**
4. **Drugs:** Phenytoin, carbamazepine, allopurinol, iron dextran
   Serum sickness
5. **Miscellaneous:** Kawasaki, amyloidosis, sinus histiocytosis, etc.

PYREXIA OF UNKNOWN ORIGIN (PUO)

Main Types

1. Classical PUO: PUO in non-compromised individual
2. Nosocomial PUO: Fever that develops in hospital and remains undiagnosed after 3 days investigation
3. Neutropenic PUO: Neutrophil <500/mm^3
4. HIV-associated PUO.

Causes

Infections

1. **Specific infections:**
   Bacterial: TB, Strep., Staph., *Brucella*, typhoid, tularemia
   Viral: Infectious mononucleosis, cytomegalovirus, dengue, HIV
   Fungal: Histoplasmosis, coccidioidomycosis
   Protozoal: Amebiasis, kala azar, toxoplasmosis, filariasis, trichinellosis
   Spirochetal: Syphilis, rat bite, relapsing, leptospirosis
   Others: Rickettsial, Q fever, psittacosis, mycoplasma
2. **Localized pus:** Abscess, sinusitis, mastoiditis, bronchiectasis, etc.
3. **Suppurative:**
   Itis: Cystitis, phlebitis, diverticulitis
   Inflamed piles
   Inflammatory bowel disease.

Non-infection

Allergic (hypersensitivity) reaction
Blood disease: Leukemia
Connective tissue dis.: SLE, temporal arteritis, systemic vasculitides

Dermal: Pemphigus, bullous dermatosis
Endocrine: Hyperthyroidism, pheochromocytoma
Factitious fever
Growths: **H**epatoma
Hypernephroma
Heart (Atrial) myxoma
Hidden: Retroperitoneal
Heat disorders
Inherited (and metabolic)
Infarction
Iatrogenic: Drug-induced
Injury

Investigations

Initial

- Chest radiograph
- Count: WBC total, dif.
- C-reactive protein
- Creatinine and electrolytes
- Urine analysis
- LFTs.

Later

- Suspected SBE: ECHO, blood culture
- Headache: Temporal artery biopsy, CT scan
- TB: Sputum culture, bone marrow and liver biopsy
- Hematuria, renal impairment: Renal ultrasono (renal cell Ca)

- Antineutrophilic cytoplasmic antibodies (vasculitis)
- Injecting drug misuse, 'high risk' sexual contacts: HIV antibody, hepatitis B and C serology.

CIGARETTE SMOKING

Harmful Effects

Angina. Amblyopia
Buerger's disease (TAO)
Carcinoma

Stomach	Bronchus
Esophagus	Bladder

Duodenal ulcer
Extrasystoles
Fetal growth restricted.

MAIN PROBLEMS OF INCREASING AGE

Instability	Incontinence
Immobility	Intellectual impairment.

STEROID SIDE-EFFECTS

Atrophy of skin and ms.
Bruising
Cataracts
Diabetes
E (**Oe**) dema

Fracture (Osteoporosis)
Gain in weight
High BP.

ALCOHOLISM

Acute Intoxication

Blood Ethanol (mg/L)	
<500	Talkativeness
500–1000	Inebriation **I**ncoherent speech **I**nstability (emotional) **I**ncoordination **I**mpaired sensation
1000–5000	Intoxication **A**taxia **B**lurred (or double vision) **C**oma. **C**onvulsions **D**ecreased sensation **E**(I)ncoordination
>5000	Very severe intoxication Coma Hypothermia Hyporeflexia Resp. depression.

Chronic Alcoholism

Hepatobiliary and Pancreatic

Hepatomegaly: Fatty liver, alcoholic hepatitis and fibrosis

Acute and chronic relapsing pancreatitis.

Nervous System

Nutritional deficiencies—Wernicke-Korsakoff, pellagra

Tobacco-alcohol amblyopia.

Others

Cerebral dementia

Central pontine myelinolysis

Fetal alcohol syndrome

Peripheral nervous system: Sensory, motor and mixed neuropathy

Autonomic neuropathy.

Musculoskeletal

Myopathy	Gout
Osteopenia	Avascular necrosis

Genitourinary

Renal disease: IgA nephropathy, renal tubular acidosis.

Reproductive Disorders

Men—Testicular atrophy, impotence

Women—Amenorrhea, subfertility, recurrent abortions, fetal damage.

Cardiovascular

Cardiomyopathy including dysrhythmias

Hypertension

Myocardial infarction.

Respiratory

Chronic bronchitis

Malignancy

Asthma.

Dermatological

Skin stigmata of liver disease

Infections—Bacterial, fungal, viral

Psoriasis

Discoid eczema

Nutritional deficiencies (including pellagra).

Gastrointestinal

Mouth: Periodontal disease and caries

Oral infections. Leukoplakia and malignancy

Esophagus: Acid regurgitation, malignancy

Stomach: Gastritis. Hematemesis

Small bowel: Enteropathy. Malabsorption
Colon: Malignancy.

Hematological

RBCs—Macrocytosis. Anemia from blood loss
WBCs—Neutropenia, lymphopenia
Platelets—Thrombocytopenia.

MULTISYSTEM DISORDERS

Systemic Lupus Erythematosus

Etiology

Immunological factors
Inherited (genetic) factors
Infection: Viral
Iatrogenic: Hydralazine, procainamide, quinidine, phenytoin, isoniazid, chlorpromazine.

Clinical Features

Arthralgia
Blood changes: Leukopenia, hemolytic anemia
CNS: Neuropathy, psychosis, fits
Dermal: Butterfly rash on face
Effusion (Pleural, pericardial). Endocarditis
Fever
Glomerulonephritis
Hematologic disorder: Hemolytic anemia, thrombocytopenia
Immunology: Positive LE cell phenomenon.

Diagnosis

ANA +ve in more than 95%.

Management

Cox-2 inhibitors (or other NSAIDs)
Chloroquine (Hydroxy)
Corticosteroids
Cytotoxic agents.

SYSTEMIC VASCULITIDES

Large Vessel

- **Giant cell arteritis**
  Arteritis (Classical temporal)
  Blindness (may occur suddenly)
  Claudication (of jaw or intermittent)
  Diplopia (and periorbital pain) due to intracranial vasculitis
- **Takayasu's arteritis**
  Arthralgia
  Aortic arch syndrome
  Aortic descending syndrome
  Arms variation in BP (>10 mm Hg)
  Audible bruit over subclavian artery
- **Polymyalgia rheumatica**
  Age: 60–70
  Bilateral shoulder pain and stiffness (also pelvic)

Constitutional symptoms
Dramatic response to corticosteroids
ESR (and CRP) raised.

Medium Vessel

- **Polyarteritis nodosa**
  Pyrexia
  Pressure (High BP)
  Pains (in joints and ms.)
  Peripheral neuritis
  Polyarteritis
  Purpura
  Pleural effusion
  Pulmonary infiltrates
  Proteinuria (and hematuria)
- **Churg-Strauss syndrome**
  Asthma
  Blood eosinophilia
  C(S)systemic vasculitis (involving 2 or more extra-pulmonary organs).

Kawasaki Disease

Diagnosis: 5 of following 6—
Fever ± 5 days' duration
Conjunctival congestion
Changes to lips (fissure) and oral cavity
Changes to peripheral extremities (red palms and soles, edema)

Cutaneous rash
Cervical lymph nodes swollen (often unilateral).

Small Vessel Vasculitis

Wegener's Granulomatosis

Triad of:
Upper resp. tract lesions
Pulmonary disease
Glomerulonephritis.

Henoch-Schönlein Purpura

Arthralgia
Bleeding: Bloody diarrhea, pulmonary hemorrhage
Cutaneous rash (buttocks and lower limbs) and GN.

Polymyositis and Dermatomyositis

DERMAL
Dermal: Heliotrope discoloration
Eyelid edema
Raynaud's
Muscle weakness (Pharyngeal, shoulder, hip)
Articular pains
Lung fibrosis.

CARCINOID SYNDROME

Abdominal cramps
Bluish discoloration of skin and mucous membrane

Cardiac involvement
Diarrhea
Emesis
Flushing (episodic).

MARFAN'S SYNDROME

Arachnodactyly
Build asthenic
Cardiac lesions (AR, MR)
Dislocation of lens
E(I)nstability of joints
Funnel-shaped chest.

SJÖGREN'S SYNDROME

Dry eyes (KCS)
Dry mouth (xerostomia)
Diverse manifestations: Arthritis, vasculitis, renal involvement. Rarely lymphoma.

POEMS SYNDROME

Polyneuropathy
Organomegaly
Endocrinopathy
M proteins
Skin changes.

LEOPARD SYNDROME

Lentigines
ECG conduction defects
Ocular hypertelorism
Pulmonary stenosis
Abnormalities of genitalia
Retardation of growth
Deafness (sensorineural).

ANTIPHOSPHOLIPID ANTIBODY SYNDROME

- **A**bortions recurrent
- **B**lood vessel disease: Thrombosis—
  Arterial: TIAs, arterial occlusion
  Venous: DVT, renal vein, Budd-Chiari syndrome
- Others: All Cs
  Cardiac: Heart valve disease
  Chorea
  Cytopenia (Thrombo)
  Convulsions (Epilepsy)
  Cord (Myelopathy)
  Crania (hemi)
  Cutaneous (livedo reticularis)
  Catastrophic syndrome: Widespreaded organ failure including ARDS.

SYSTEMIC SCLEROSIS

Clinical Features

- **Limited cutaneous systemic sclerosis**
  Long history of antecedent Raynaud's with recurrent digital ulceration. Also esophageal dysmotility
- **Diffuse cutaneous systemic sclerosis**
  Presence of sclerosis proximal to elbows and knees or affecting the trunk
- **Systemic sclerosis sine scleroderma**
  Typical vascular features of systemic sclerosis with visceral complications like lung fibrosis, hypertensive renal crisis or severe bowel involvement.

TURNER'S SYNDROME

Sexual: Amenorrhea (primary)
Sexual infantilism

Skeletal: Short stature
Shield-like chest
Short metacarpal
Short neck
Scoliosis
Small mandible
Salmon (fish-like) mouth

Soft tissues:	Webbing of neck
	Lymphedema
Skin:	Small nipples
	Pigmented nevi
CVS:	Aortic stenosis
	Bicuspid aortic valve
	Coarctation
Renal:	Rotation of kidneys, duplex ureters, etc.

PORPHYRIAS

Acute Porphyrias

Common Features

All three autosomal dominant
All three often precipitated by drugs
All three potentially life-threatening.

Types

Intermittent	Variegate
Hereditary coproporphyria	Plumbo.

Clinical Features: 4 Ps

Pains in abdomen
Polyneuropathy
Psychosis
Pink urine.

Precipitating Factors

Pregnancy
Alcohol
Infection
Drugs

  Anticonvulsants (Porphobilinogen)
  Barbiturates
  Contraceptives (oral)
  Diazine (Sulfa)

Note: Acute porphyria should be considered if—
Unexplained peripheral neuropathy
Unexplained abdominal pain
Unexplained neurosis and psychosis.

Non-acute or Cutaneous Porphyrias

- Cutaneous hepatic
- Erythropoietic
- Congenital (Rare).

Clinical Features

Characteristic skin lesions and photosensitivity.

AMYLOIDOSIS

Classification

Localized Amyloidosis

1. **Senile:** Deposits in heart, joints

2. **Cerebral:** Alzheimer's disease, cerebral amyloid angiopathy, prion disease
   Subacute spongiform encephalopathy (Creutzfeldt-Jakob disease)
3. **Hemodialysis associated**
4. **Endocrine:** In AUPD organs, islets of Langerhans
5. Isolated massive nodular deposits in skin, lung, urogenital tract.

Systemic Amyloidosis

Clinical features:

Renal:	Proteinuria	
	Nephrotic syndrome	
	Nephrogenic diabetes insipidus	
	Hypertension	
Respiratory:	Dyspnea	Stridor
	Hemoptysis	Cough
Cardiac:	**A**rrhythmias	
	Biventricular 'diastolic' failure	
	Const. pericarditis (mimics)	
	Decubital (postural) hypotension	
	E(I)schemic heart disease	
Skin:	Alopecia, purpura, plaques, bullous eruptions	
Musculoskeletal:	Like RA	
	Muscle infiltration	
	Dialysis arthropathy syndrome	

Gastrointestinal tract:	**C**onstipation
	Dysphagia
	Diarrhea
	Enlarged tongue
	Faulty absorption
	GI hemorrhage
	Hepatosplenomegaly
	Intestinal obst., perforation
Nervous system:	Peripheral neuropathy
	Autonomic neuropathy
	Carpal tunnel syndrome
	Enlarged peripheral ns.
Miscellaneous:	**A**denopathy. **A**drenal involvement.
	Bleeding (with normal clotting factors)
	C(S)icca syndrome—Dry eyes, mouth
	Deficiency of factors IX, X
	Enlarged thyroid.

METABOLIC ENCEPHALOPATHIES

Hypoglycemia
Hyponatremia
Hypoxia
Hypercapnia
Hypo- or hyperosmolar states

Hepatic (and uremic) encephalopathy
High grade (severe)
Peripheral circulatory failure.

METABOLIC BONE DISEASE

1. Osteoporosis—Thin bone
2. Osteosclerosis—Thick bone
3. Osteomalacia—Rickets
4. Osteitis fibrosa.

Osteoporosis

Idiopathic

- **S**enile
- **I**diopathic (Juvenile or adult)
- **P**ostmenopausal.

Secondary

Arthritis (Rheumatoid)
Bed rest (Immobilization)
Carcinoma: Breast, kidney, lung, thyroid. Multiple myeloma
Drugs: Glucocorticoids, heparin, thyroxine, diuretics (frusemide), cytotoxic therapy.
Endocrine: **H**ypogonadism (either sex)
Hyperadrenocorticism
Hydrocortisone (steroid) therapy
Hyperthyroidism

Fat: Obesity
Glomerulonephritis (Nephrotic syndrome)
Heart transplantation (or kidney or liver)
Heparin therapy (prolonged)
Inadequate absorption (Malabsorption).

Prevention and Treatment

Anabolic steroids
Bisphosphonates (Etidronate)
Calcium. Calcitonin
D_3 vitamin
Exercise
Fluoride (Sodium).

OSTEOMALACIA

Causes

1. **Vitamin D deficiency:**
   Deficient supply (Nutritional)
   Impaired absorption
   Failure of hydroxylation—Chronic liver disease, kidney failure
2. **Familial hypophosphatemic rickets**
3. **Multifactorial:** Anticonvulsants
4. **Uncertain pathogenesis:** Renal tubular acidosis, hypophosphatemic osteomalacia.

Clinical Features

Rickets

Costochondral prominence (Rickety rosary)
Deformity of long bones
Epiphyseal expansion at wrists
Frontal bossing
Generalized muscle weakness
Hypocalcemic symptoms.

Osteomalacia in Adults

Bone pains
Fractures
Proximal myopathy
Hypocalcemic symptoms.

INBORN ERRORS OF METABOLISM

Mucopolysaccharidoses

(Hurler's, Hunter's, Maroteaux-Lamy, Morquio syndromes)
Bony abnormalities (Dysostosis multiplex)
Corneal clouding
Dementia
Enlarged liver, spleen.

Inborn Errors of Carbohydrate Metabolism

Glycogen Storage Disease

Von Gierke

Hepatosplenomegaly	**H**yperlipidemia
Hypotension	**H**yperuricemia
Hypoglycemia	**H**(O)besity

Galactosemia

Anorexia
Acidosis
Ascites (with hepatomegaly and jaundice)

McArdle's disease

Failure of breakdown of glycogen to glucose due to deficiency of myophosphorylase.
Pentosuria and essential fructosuria.

AMINOACIDURIAS

Maple Syrup Urine Disease

Phenylketonuria

Mental retardation
Depigmentation of skin and hair
Seizures.

Homocystinuria

Same as Marfan's plus mental retardation and fits.

Alkaptonuria
Arthritis
Black urine
Ochronosis.

IMMUNODEFICIENCY DISEASES

Main groups at risk of infections:

1. **Immunodeficiency (primary)**—Congenital defects of antibody production, e.g. hypogammaglobulinemia or of T cell function, (e.g. DiGeorge's syndrome)
2. **Immunologically compromised patients**—AIDS, malnutrition, burns, hematological malignancies
3. **Immunosuppressed patients**—Corticosteroid or cytotoxic therapy, splenectomy, kidney transplant.

Autoimmune Diseases in Man

Liver:	**A**lcoholic liver disease
	Biliary cirrhosis
	Cryptogenic cirrhosis
	Drug sensitivity (hepatic)
	Hepatitis and chronic active hepatitis.
GI:	**A**trophic gastritis
	Bowel disease (inflammatory)
	Celiac disease

Renal:	Glomerulonephritis	
Endocrine:	Thyroiditis	Diabetes
	Thyrotoxicosis	Hypoparathyroid
	Addison's (idio.)	Polyendocrine syndrome
CNS:	Myasthenia	
	MS, GB syndrome	
Skin:	Eczema. Vitiligo	
	Psoriasis	Leprosy
	Alopecia areata	Pyoderma gangrenosum
Others:	Goodpasture's syndrome	
	Serum sickness (acute), AIDS	

Congenital Immunodeficiencies

1. Antibodies: Hypogammaglobulinemia (X-linked) IgG, IgA, IgM deficiencies
2. T cells: Thymic aplasia, chronic mucocutaneous candidiasis
3. B cells, T cells: Wiskott-Aldrich syndrome, enzyme deficiencies
4. Phagocytes: Chronic granulomatous disease, lazy leukocytes
5. Complement: C_2 or C_4 deficiency.

Immunotherapies

Some therapeutic agents

Agents	*Indications*
• **Monoclonal antibodies**	
Abciximab	Prevention of restenosis postpercutaneous coronary intervention
Infliximab	Moderate to severe Crohn's disease. RA not responding to methotrexate
Rituximab	Relapsed or refractory low-grade or follicular NHL
• **Fusion proteins**	
Etanercept	Moderate-to-severe RA Polyarticular juvenile RA
• **Soluble cytokine receptor**	
Anakinra	Moderate-to-severe RA
• **Cytokines**	
F-N-α	Chronic HVC infection, AIDS-related sarcoma, hairy cell leukemia
IL-2	Renal cell Ca, metastatic melanoma

- **Erythropoietin** Anemia, CKF
- G-CSF, GM-CSF } Reversal of neutropenia after chemotherapy, radiation therapy or both.

GENETICS

Major Groups

1. **Chromosome Anomalies**
   Autosome Anomalies
   - Down's syndrome 47, + 12
     Affable and affectionate
     Brachycephaly, **B**rushfield's spots
     Canthic (epi) folds
     Dwarfism
     Ears small
     Fingers short and stubby
   - Patau's syndrome 47, + 13
     Arhinencephaly
     Bilateral hydronephrosis (often)
     Cleft lip and palate
     Deafness
     Ears low set. **E**yes small
     Fingers: Polydactyly

- Edward's syndrome 47, + 18
  Clenched overlapping fingers
  Dolichocephaly
  Ears low set, malformed
  Feet: "Rocker bottom"
  Gnathia (Micrognathia)
  Hypertonicity.

Sex Chromosome Anomalies

- Turner's syndrome 45, X: WASP
  Webbing of neck
  Amenorrhea
  Short stature (infantilism)
  Pigmented nevi
- Klinefelter's syndrome 47, XXY
  Decreased: Size of testis, pubis-heel ratio
  Eunuchoid features
  Fatty tendency
  Gynecomastia
- XYY syndrome 47, XYY
  Increased height
  Minor mental retardation
- Triple X syndrome 47, XXX
  Increased tendency to psychosis
  Normal physical features.

2. Single Gene Defects

AD	*AR*	*XLR*	*Variable*
Achondropl.	**A**lbinism	**A**nderson-Fabry	**R**etini. pigment.
Bourneville's disease	**β**-Thalas.	**B**lood dis. (Hemoph.)	Ehlers-Danlos
Chorea (Hunting)	**C**(S)ickle cell anemia	**C**horeo-athetoid, self muti (Lesch-Nyhan)	**P**olycystic kidneys
Dystrophia myotonia	**D**ystrophy (Scaphum) Dysplasia (thoracic)	**D**iabetes (Ins.)	**A**taxia (spino-cerebellar)
E(I)nterm. porphy.	**E**nzyme dis. (Phenylketo.)	**D**ystrophy (Duchenne)	Ichthyosis
Facioscapulo hum. dys.	**F**ibrosis (cystic)	**E**nzyme def. (G6PD)	Deafness
Generalized neurofibro.	**G**alactosemia	**F**eminization	Dystrophies muscular
Hypercholes.	Tay Sachs	Menke's syn.	Mucopoly-sacch
Int. (colonic) polypi			
Marfan's			

3. Multifactorial diseases

Congenital

CNS defects (Neural tube)

Congenital dislocation of hip

Cleft lip

Cardiac disease

C(S)tenosis: Pyloric

Acquired

Abnormal behavior (Psychoses)
BP rise
Coronary heart disease
Duodenal ulcer
Diabetes mellitus
Epilepsy.

TYPES OF IMMUNE REACTIONS

Anaphylaxis	Anaphylactic
Causes	Cytotoxic hypersensitivity Transfusion reaction Drug reaction—Hemolytic anemia
Immediate	Immune complex reaction, e.g. Serum reaction
Collapse	Cell-mediated hypersensitivity, e.g. tuberculin reaction.

INFECTIONS TRANSMITTED FROM ANIMALS

Perfume	Psittacosis
Abolishes	Anthrax
Lousy	Leptospirosis
Body	Brucellosis
Odor	Orf.

TREPONEMAL DISEASES AFFECTING MAN

Syphilis
Pinta
Yaws.

DYSLIPIDEMIAS

1. Primary or inherited
2. Secondary.

Causes

Common

Alcohol excess
Bad kidneys (Kidney failure)
Cholestatic jaundice, e.g. biliary cirrhosis
Diabetes mellitus
Endocrine: Hypothyroidism
Fat (Obesity)
Glomerulonephritis (Nephrotic syndrome).

Less Common

Amyloidosis (primary)
Blood disease: Myeloma
Contraceptive (oral)
Drugs: Thiazide diuretics, beta-blockers
Exercise lack
Gammaglobulinemia (Hyper)
Hyperuricemia (gout).

Manifestations of Dyslipidemia

1. **Xanthalesmata:** Cholesterol deposits at inner margins of eyelids.
2. **Xanthomata:**
   Tendon—Hypercholesterolemia
   Palmar—Type III hyperlipoproteinemia
   Eruptive—Hypertriglyceridemia
3. **Lipemia retinalis:** Chylomicrons or Triglycerides
4. **Premature coronary artery disease:** All hyperlipidemias except chylomicrons and VLDL
5. **Pancreatitis:** Chylomicrons and VLDL.

METABOLIC SYNDROME (SYNDROME X)

Features

Endocrine and Biochemical Abnormalities

At least 3 of—

- Abdominal obesity (waist circumference >80 cm in males >90 cm in females
- High triglyceride levels (>150 m/dL)
- High fasting glucose
- Hypertension S/D 130/85 mm Hg
- Reduced HDL cholesterol level.

Other Pathological Conditions

- Type 2 diabetes mellitus
- Coronary heart disease
- Polycystic ovary syndrome

- Central fat distribution
- Morbid obesity
- Stress and depression
- Hypertension
- Non-alcoholic steatohepatitis
- Sleep-disordered breathing
- Chronic kidney disease
- Erectile dysfunction.

DISORDERS OF WATER AND ELECTROLYTE METABOLISM

Water

Excess

ADH inappropriate secretion
Beer drinking (excessive)
Compulsive water drinking
Drugs: Carbamazepine
Excessive IV fluids
Failure of kidneys: Acute or severe chronic with dialysis
Glucocorticoid deficiency: Addison's disease, anterior pituitary failure
Hypothalamic lesions
Irrigation: Total bowel or colorectal.

Deficiency: 5 Ds

Dearth of water
Drowsiness
Dysphagia (severe)
Diabetes mellitus or insipidus
Diuresis

Sodium

Hypernatremia

1. **Hypovolemia**
   - Dermal losses: Excessive sweating
   - Diarrhea, prolonged vomiting
   - Diabetes mellitus
   - Diuretic therapy (excessive)
   - Due to renal loss:
     - Addison's disease, hypoaldosteronism
     - Renal salt wasting: Chronic pyelonephritis, renal calculus disease
     - Excessive ultrafiltration: Hemoperitoneal dialysis.
2. **Hypervolemia**
   Iatrogenic: Hypertonic saline, tube feeding
3. **Euvolemia:** Fever, diabetes insipidus, hyperventilation, mechanical ventilation.

Hyponatremia

1. **Excessive loss**

Skin:	Excessive sweating
GI tract:	Vomiting, diarrhea, fistula
Renal:	Diabetes mellitus
	Diuretic therapy
	Deficiency of mineralocorticoids
	Depletion of salt (Renal salt wasting).

2. **Excessive ultrafiltration by dialysis.**

POTASSIUM

Hyperkalemia

1. **Excessive intake:** Parenteral
2. **Decreased excretion:**
   Addison's disease
   Angiotensin-converting enzyme inhibitors
   Acute oliguric (or chronic) kidney failure
   Amiloride (and other K-sparing diuretics).
3. **Redistribution**
   Catabolic states
   Acidosis
   Tissue damage.

Hypokalemia

1. **Decreased intake:** Oral (starvation), parenteral.
2. **Increased excretion:**
   GI: Diarrhea, vomiting, drainage, purgative abuse
   Renal: Diuretics (loop, thiazide), diuretic phase of ARF, renal tubular acidosis
3. **Redistribution:** Insulin. Alkalosis. Rapid cell proliferation.

Clinical Features

Hyperkalemia	**Hypokalemia**
Generalized m. weakness	M. weakness
	Tetany

Cardiac arrest	Arrhythmias
	Polyuria
	Paralytic ileus
ECG: Tall T	Tall U
Wide QRS	Wide PR
Absent P	Absent U.

ACID-BASE BALANCE

Normal: Arterial pH 7.35–7.45
$PaCO_2$ 35–40 mm Hg

Disorder	*Causes*	*Primary changes*
Metabolic acidosis (Acid production, excretion or metabolism)	Diabetic keto., lactic acidosis, alcohol poisoning, kidney failure	$\uparrow H^+$ $-HCO_3^-$
Metabolic alkalosis (Loss or removal of acid)	Gastric aspirate Vomiting Excess alkali	$\downarrow H^+$ $-HCO_3^-$
Respiratory acidosis (Excess CO_2 retention)	Ventilatory failure (e.g. chronic bronchitis, anoxia, drugs)	$\uparrow H^+$ $-PCO_2$ $-HCO_3^-$

Respiratory alkalosis	Inappropriate hyperventilation (e.g. sustained hypercapnia with cerebral irritation)	↓H^+ -PCO_2 -HCO_3^-

Mixed Disorders

Respiratory and metabolic acidosis in hypoventilated hypoxic patient.

Respiratory alkalosis and metabolic acidosis in salicylate poisoning.

Relation Between pH and $PaCO_2$

Guidelines

For every increase in $PaCO_2$ of 20 mm Hg (2.6 kPa) above normal the pH falls by 0.1.

For every decrease in of $PaCO_2$ of 10 mm Hg (1.3 kPa) below normal the pH rises by 0.1. Any change in pH outside these parameters is therefore metabolic in origin.

Tips for Respiratory Alkalosis

Normal pH 7.40
Normal $PaCO_2$ 40 mm Hg in pure metabolic acidosis, if pH falls to say 7.22, $PaCO_2$ would be 22, but if $PaCO_2$

is say 15, it indicates superimposed primary resp. alkalosis.

Anion Gap

Organisms exist in a state of electroneutrality with major and minor cations balanced by similar anions. The anion gap is a disparity between concentrations of major plasma cations and anions routinely measured—normally sodium, chloride, and bicarbonate.

Anion gap = $Na^+ - (Cl + HCO_3)$.

Cystic Fibrosis: LIP

Lung disease (chronic)
Infertility
Pancreatitis.

SOME SYMPTOMS AND SIGNS

Acanthosis Nigricans: HOME

Hereditary
Obesity
Malignancy: Adenocarcinoma
Endocrine: Diabetes, Acromegaly, Cushing's, Polycystic ovary syn., Hypothyroidism, Addison's disease

Bromhidrosis

E(A)pocrine: Axillary
Eccrine: Keratinogenic
Endocrine: Metabolic
Exogenous: Foods, drugs, chemicals
Plantar
Intertriginous
Heritable amiauavios

Calf Muscle Hypertrophy

Inherited (Genetically determined)—Duchenne, **B**ecker, Charcot-Marie-Tooth.
Inflammatory—Myositis ossificans
Infection (Parasitic)—Trichinosis, cysticercosis
Injury—Tendon rupture
Infiltration—Amyloidosis
Endocrine—Acromegaly, hypothyroidism.

Carotenemia

Anorexia nervosa
Beta-carotene therapy (for erythropoietic porphyria)
Carrot eating (excessive)
Diabetes mellitus
Endocrine: Hypothyroidism.

Carpal Tunnel Syndrome: CARPAL

Compression (of ulnar nerve)
Acromegaly
Rheumatoid arthritis (Also osteo)
Pregnancy
Amyloid
Lone (idiopathic).

Cholinergic Drugs

Adverse Effects: DUMBEL

Diarrhea
Urinary incontinence
Miosis
Bradycardia, **B**ronchospasm
Emesis
Lacrimation.

Dehydration

Absorption failure
Burns
Cathartics and diuretics
Diarrhea and vomiting
Excessive perspiration
Fluid intake minimal.

Epiglottitis: 4 Ds

Dysphagia	**D**rooling
Dysphonia	**D**istress (Resp.).

Erythema Nodosum

Immunological disease: Rheumatic fever, Behcet's
Infection: Streptococcal, tuberculosis, leprosy.
Viral and chlamydial infection, lymphogr. venereum, toxoplasmosis, brucellosis
Infiltration: Sarcoidosis
Inflammatory bowel disease
Iatrogenic: Drugs, e.g. Sulfonamides, contraceptive pill
Idiopathic.

Fatigue (Chronic)

Psychogenic: Anxiety states, depression
Physiological: Insomnia, overwork
Pathological:

- **A**lcoholism
- **B**lood disease: Anemia, leukemia, lymphoma
- **C**hest disease: Chronic lung or cardiovascular disease
- **D**rugs: Steroids, barbiturates
- **E**ndocrine: Diabetes, hypothyroidism, Addison's disease, thyrotoxicosis

Fevers (prolonged)
Growths (malignant)
Hepatic disease: Chronic hepatitis, cirrhosis
Infections: Tuberculosis
Joint (or neuromuscular disease)
Kidney disease: Uremia.

Familial Dyslipidemia: Triad of TAX

Tendon xanthomata
Xanthelasma
Arcus corneae.

Fever with Chills

- Bacterial infection including pneumonia, IE
- Malaria
- Kala azar
- Meningococcal meningitis
- Acute pyelonephritis
- Erysipelas
- Allergic reaction: IV drugs, blood products
- Weil's disease.

Fever in Cancer Patient

Infection: Septicemia, intermittent bacteremias (esp. from central line, occult localized infections, e.g.

cryptococcal meningitis, viremia (esp. CMV, e.g. following marrow transplant)

Iatrogenic: Bleomycin, L-Asparaginase, interferon, transfusions

Incidental to primary disease: Lymphoma, retroperitoneal tumors (e.g. renal cell Ca), metastatic liver disease (tumor necrosis).

Hiccough

Abdomen: Liver or subphrenic abscess, intestinal obst., peritonitis

Brain: e.g. TB meningitis, tumor

Chest: Mediastinal tumor, aortic aneurysm

Diabetes or toxic conditions, e.g. uremia, alcoholism, severe systemic infection

E(I)diopathic: No known cause

Functional: After bouts of laughter, hysterical.

Hypertrichosis

Congenital (Hereditary) Disorders

Hurler's syndrome, lipoatrophy, Porphyria.

Acquired

Anorexia nervosa

Bad nutrition

Cerebral disturbance, e.g. after head injury

Dermatomyositis

Endocrine: Hypothyroidism, pretibial myxedema
Iatrogenic: Streptomycin, corticosteroids, diphenylhydantoin, penicillamine, psoralens, diazoxide, minoxidil, cyclosporin.

Iodine Deficiency Disorders

Fetus	Neonates	Infant/Child/ Adolescent	Adult
Spontaneous abortions Stillbirths Congenital anomalies Increased perinatal and infant mortality	Goiter Overt or subclinical hypothyroidism	Goiter subclinical or overt hypothyroidism Mental retardation Retarded physical development Increased susceptibility of thyroid gland to radiation	Goiter and its complication Hypothyroidism Mental retardation Decreased fertility Spontaneous hyperthyroidism in elderly Increased susceptibility of thyroid to nuclear radiation

Kyphoscoliosis

Arthritis (Rheumatoid)
Bone disease: Paget's
Congenital
D vitamin deficiency (Rickets)
E(I)diopathic
Friedreich's ataxia and other neurological disease, e.g. syringomyelia.

Leg Ulcers

Vascular Disease

- **Venous:** Venous thrombosis
- **Arterial:** Atherosclerosis, hypertension, IAO, cholesterol emboli
- **Vasculitis:** Small, medium and large vessel
- **Neuropathy:** Neuropathic DM, tabes, syringomyelia, peripheral nerve lesions
- **Metabolic:** DM, gout, Gaucher's disease, calciphylaxis
- **Hematologic:** Sickle cell anemia, hereditary spherocytosis, thalassemia, dysproteinemias
- **Trauma:** Cold, burns, radiation-induced dermatitis
- **Neoplastic:** Basal cell Ca, Kaposi's sarcoma, lymphoma
- **Infections:** Bacterial, fungal, protozoal

- **Specific dermatoses:** Necrobiosis lipoidica, pyoderma gangrenosum
- **Genetic:** Klinefelter's syndrome.

Loss of Memory

Alcoholism
B vitamin deficiency—B_1, B_{12}, nicotinic acid
Cerebral atrophy, tumor
Disseminated sclerosis
Endocrine—Hypothyroidism
Functional (Hysterical)
GPI (and meningovascular syphilis)
Huntington's chorea
Iatrogenic—Sedative drugs, ECT.

Lump in Left Iliac Fossa

Adenopathy (iliac)
Bowel (fecal) lumps
Crohn's disease
Diverticulitis
Ectopic kidney
Follicular cyst (ovarian)
Growth.

Lump in Right Iliac Fossa

Appendicular abscess

Bowel inflammation: Crohn's
Carcinoid
Dropped (ectopic) kidney
E(I)nfection: Ameboma, actinomycosis, schistosomiasis
Female disorder: Tubal pregnancy, ovarian tumor
Growth: Carcinoma cecum
Hypertrophic ileocecal TB
Intussusception.

Oculogyric Crisis

Postencephalitic
Parkinsonism
Petit mal epilepsy
Phenothiazines.

Edema

Generalized: Anasarca

Anemia (and hypoproteinemia)
Beriberi
Constrictive pericarditis
Dropsy (epidemic)
Endocrine (myxedema)
Failure (CHF)
Glomerulonephritis (nephrosis)
Hepatic disease: Cirrhosis, portal hypertension
Iatrogenic: Steroids, nifedipine, amlodipine.

Localized (Or Unilateral)

Inflammatory: Cellulitis
Insufficiency: Lymphatic—Operation, irradiation, congenital absence, lymphoma
Idiopathic
Inherited: Milroy's disease
Insect bites and stings.

Orthostatic Hypotension

Abnormal venous pooling, e.g. prolonged standing, varicose veins
Bed rest (prolonged)
Chronic idiopathic orthostatic hypotension
Decreased vasomotor activity: Peripheral neuropathy (diabetic), syringomyelia, Shy-Drager syndrome.
Drugs: Hypotensive therapy, tranquillizers, levodopa
Endocrine: Hypopituitarism, Addison's disease
Fluid depletion.

Pallor

Hemolytic anemia
Hypothyroidism
Hypopituitarism
Hypoproteinemia, e.g. nephrosis
Heart disease: Acute infarction, tight AS or MS, acute LVF

Hypovolemic shock (also septicemic)
Hypochondriasis: Fear.

Palmar Erythema

Alcoholism, arthritis (rheumatoid)
Blood disease: Polycythemia
Collagen vascular disease: SLE
Dermal: Tinea, eczematoid dermatitis, psoriasis
Endocrine: Thyrotoxicosis, diabetes mellitus
Familial
Gestation (Pregnancy)
Hepatic disease: Hepatitis, cirrhosis
Incompetence: Mitral regurgitation.

Priapism

Local Causes

Perineal trauma or infection. Tumors.

General Causes

Abuse of: Alcohol, marijuana
Blood diseases: Sickle cell disease, thalassemia, leukemia, thrombocytopenia
CNS disease: Cerebral vascular accident. Sp. cord injury
Drug therapy: Chlorpromazine, haloperidol, hydralazine, reserpine, diazepam, anticoagulants
E(I)diopathic
Failure: Kidney failure.

Protein-losing Enteropathy

Intestinal: Inflammatory bowel disease, celiac disease, sprue

Infiltration: Ca stomach, colon

IVC obstruction. Also constrictive pericarditis, cirrhosis.

Infiltrate: Whipple's disease, eosinophilic enteritis.

Pruritus (Generalized)

Systemic Causes

Allergy
Blood diseases: Polycythemia, anemia, Hodgkin's
Collagen diseases: SLE
Drugs: Opiates, belladonna
Endocrine: Diabetes, hypothyroidism
Functional: Psychosis
Gestation (Pregnancy)
HIV
Helminths
Jaundice (obstructive)
Kidney failure
Liver disease: Primary biliary cirrhosis, chronic liver failure
Malignancy
Neurological: Multiple sclerosis
Old age
Parasitic infections: Trichinosis, schistosomiasis.

Raynaud's Syndrome

Raynaud's disease plus:

Arterial disease: Embolism, AO, costoclavicular syndrome

Blood diseases: polycythemia vera, paroxysmal cold hemoglobinuria

Collagen disorders: RA, Sjogren's, PAN, dermato/polymyositis, systemic sclerosis

Developmental: Syringomyelia

Ergot

F(ph)ysical: Vibration, cold.

Rectal Bleeding

Antibiotic use (Pseudomembranous colitis)

Bowel disease (Inflammatory)

Cancer (also polyps)

Diverticular colitis

E(I)schemic colitis

Fissures (and other perianal lesions)

Gay bowel syndrome

Hemorrhoids

Irradiation proctitis.

Red Face

Autonomic (vasomotor) instability

Birth mark (port wine stain)

Carcinoid syndrome
Drugs: Steroids
Epidermal: Dermatitis—atopic, contact, seborrheic. Rosacea, psoriasis, erysipelas, lupus, dermatomyositis
Female menopause
Growths (Mediastinal).

Rhinitis

Allergic
Bacterial infection
Chronic non-specific (NARES syndrome)
Drugs, e.g. decongestant nasal sprays
Endocrine: Diabetes, hypothyroidism
Foreign body
Growths: Polyps, neoplasms
Hypersensitive response of nasal mucosa (Vasomotor rhinitis).

Rings Around Cornea: ABCs

Arcus senilis
Band keratopathy
C(K)ayser Fleischer ring
Cystinosis
Chloroquine crystals after prolonged use (e.g. discoid lupus erythematosus).

Trismus

Tetanus
Tonsillar (peri) abscess
Tonsillitis acute
Temporomandibular arthritis
Tooth impacted
Tetany (sometimes)
Transient: Drug-induced dyskinesia
Terical (Hysterical).

Weight Loss

Anorexia nervosa
Bad absorption (Malabsorption syndrome)
Cancer
Depression
Endocrine: Diabetes, thyrotoxicosis, hypoadrenalism
Fevers: Tuberculosis
GI causes: Esophageal lesions, gastric ulcer.

Notes

Aortic Dissection: MATCH

Marfan syndrome
Accelerated hypertension
Trauma
Coarctation of aorta
Hypertension in pregnancy.

Acute Aortic Regurgitation

Annulo-aortic ectasia
Blunt chest wall trauma
Cusp (myxomatous) tear
Dissection of aorta
Endocarditis of aortic valve.

Dyspnea of Sudden Onset: MAPS

Myocardial infarction
Aortic dissection
Pulmonary embolism
Spontaneous pneumothorax
Sinus of Valsalva rupture

Effects of LA Myxoma: VICE

Valvular obstruction
Inflammatory features: Anemia, leukocytosis, high ESR
Constitutional symptoms: Fever, arthralgia, weight loss
Embolism (peripheral).

Pericardial Effusion: Causes

Infection: TB
Infiltration: Metastasis
Injury
Iatrogenic: Drugs, irradiation
Immune (Auto): RA, SLE
Infarction.

Insidious Headache

Subdural hematoma
Sinusitis (chronic)
Sinus thrombosis (venous)
Senile (giant cell) arteritis
Stress (Tension) headache
Sinus/pharynx Ca.

Acute Onset Headache

Abscess
BP rise
Cluster headache

Dessection (carotid vertebral artery)
Encephalitis
Facial (Trigeminal neuralgia)
Glaucoma
Hemorrhage (SAH)
Hydrocephalus
Intracerebral hemorrhage.

RV Infarction: Suggested By

Hypotension
Distended jugular veins
Clear lung fields.

Tuberous Sclerosis or Epiloia

Epilepsy
Low intelligence
Adenoma sebaceum.

Geriatric Incontinence: DIAPERS

Delirium
Infection (UTI)
Atrophic urethritis/Vaginitis
Psychological
Pharmaceuticals
Excess urine output
Restricted mobility
Stool impaction.

Resuscitation Procedures in Newborn Infants: TABC

Temperature maintenance
Airway
Breathing
Circulation maintenance.

Raynaud's Phenomenon

Types:

1. **Primary** — Fingers → toes; Family history
2. **Secondary**

Arterial disease (obliterative)
Blood dsycrasias: Myeloproliferative disorders, hyperviscosity syndrome
Collagen vascular disease
CNS disorders, Carpal tunnel syndrome
Drug induced: Ergot, β blockers
Employment: Vibration tool injury
Environmental: Frostbite.

Clinical Features of Pheochromocytoma: PHD

Palpitation
Hypertension
Diaphoresis.

Malignant Melanoma (MM)

Asymmetrical pigmented nodule
Border irregularity
Color variability
Diameter >5 mm
Elevation irregularity.